PROSTATE REVOLUTION

THE UNDERGROUND GUIDE

TO STRONG FLOW, CURB THE URGE TO GO, AND SLEEP THROUGH THE NIGHT...

RACHAEL ROSS MD, PhD

Prostate Revolution : The Underground Guide to Flow Strong, Curb The Urge to Go Pee, & Sleep Through The Night
By Rachael Ross M.D., PhD

CONTENTS

PREFACE:

As a daughter, one of the hardest things I have had to do is watch my dad struggle with an enlarged prostate. An enlarged prostate emasculated my dad in a way that I wasn't prepared for.

He was such a kind, caring gentleman who poured love and support into anyone close to him, and I will forever be proud to say he was my dad. The last year of his life was a struggle for us both. His prostate was so large that urinating was a struggle. He would urinate sometimes without knowing it, and often, the urge was so extreme that he couldn't hold it anymore.

The last few years of his life were spent searching out bathrooms and keeping urinals in his car so he wouldn't have to stop at gas stations and fast-food restaurants to urinate. My dad waited until it was too late to get started on prostate care. He didn't want to take the medication, but he also didn't try much else. My dad was busy trying to help everyone else and didn't look after himself like he could have. He was deathly afraid of surgery, as he had every right to be because he had performed enough of them in his day to know that anything could happen.

To see the look of shame on his face as I had to help change his adult diaper, change the linen, and help him to the toilet at times was more than anyone could have prepared me for. The man I had spent so much of my life getting help from needed help from me.

As a daughter and as a physician, it was really hard for me. But it pushed me into my calling to educate men worldwide about how to prevent themselves from being in a situation like my dad's. It inspired me to begin to create a supplement that would change lives. It inspired me to do more. I hope the information in this book helps you and the men in your life that you love. Within this book, you will find nuggets of information that I designed to give you the knowledge you need to maintain a healthy prostate. After you read it, you will know exactly why and also why your doctor never told you these things about your prostate. He likely didn't know himself. This book is for you, dad!

INTRODUCTION

The Prostate is More Important Than They Tell You it Is

In the intricate tapestry of the male body, nestled deep within, lies an organ whose significance is often downplayed or, worse, ignored: the prostate. For many, it's just a word thrown around in medical conversations, accompanied by a vague understanding of its role. However, it's so much more than that.

The prostate is not just another body part; it's a cornerstone of male sexual health. It plays a pivotal role in pleasure, fertility, and overall well-being. Yet, despite its importance, it's rarely the focal point of our health conversations until something goes wrong. Why is that? Perhaps it's due to the silence shrouding male sexual health, or maybe it's the underlying biases in medical practices. The truth is, many of us have been left in the dark about the full range of what our prostate offers us, the ways to keep it healthy, and the potential risks we should be aware of.

This isn't your typical medical guidebook filled with jargon and impersonal advice. Instead, this book aims to shed light on the untold stories and secrets of the prostate that many doctors might never share with you. From its role in ecstatic pleasures to its silent signals of distress, we delve deep into understanding this critical organ like never before. Because when it comes to prostate care, what you don't know can indeed hurt you.

Whether you're reading this out of sheer curiosity, concern, or a desire for better health, by the end of this guide, you'll be equipped with knowledge that could redefine your perspective on male health. We'll challenge some widely accepted notions, debunk myths, and offer a holistic approach to prostate care, ensuring you have the tools to take control of your well-being.

The Truth about Medical Bias and the Prostate

Navigating the healthcare system can feel like walking through a labyrinth, especially when it comes to areas of the body that have historically been cloaked in taboo, like the prostate. While medical science has made monumental strides in understanding and treating numerous conditions, there remains a noticeable bias, either unintentional or by design, when it comes to addressing prostate health holistically.

For instance, why is it that many men are unaware of the prostate's function until they face a medical issue? Why does society tend to focus more on the potential problems of the prostate rather than its essential roles and proactive care? It begs the question: are we receiving a complete picture of our health from the medical community, or are critical pieces missing from the puzzle?

The unsettling truth is that certain aspects of male health, specifically concerning the prostate, often get sidelined. A potential reason could be the system's overreliance on pharmaceutical solutions or expensive, invasive procedures, which sometimes seem more like a quick fix than a long-term solution. Another potential reason prostate health isn't a focus is that without a healthy prostate, fertility is limited. If you believe that there is a conspiracy to decrease fertility worldwide, millions of enlarged prostates are one way to do just that. As you will learn, the prostate is an integral part of propelling sperm-rich semen into the vaginal canal. If the prostate is enlarged, damaged, or removed, it becomes increasingly difficult to get a partner pregnant.

It's essential to recognize that many dedicated doctors go above and beyond to provide comprehensive care to their patients. It is important to note that some doctors just don't know and are regurgitating what they have been taught. However, as a patient, knowledge is the best defense against any oversight. By understanding your body and the intricacies of the prostate, you can have better conversations with your healthcare providers, ensuring a care path tailored to your unique needs and understanding.

This book endeavors to bridge the gap by diving into the depths of prostate health, from its function in sexual pleasure to its role in fertility. I aim to equip you with the knowledge and tools to effectively advocate for yourself and your health. I want you to be able to Live Free & Go Hard in the pursuit of a healthy prostate.

CHAPTER 1:
PROSTATE - THE CENTER OF FERTILITY & UNSPOKEN DANGERS

Anatomy and Vital Role of the Prostate

Sitting at the base of the penis, positioned between the bladder and the penis and resembling the size and shape of a walnut, weighing about 20 grams, this organ might appear insignificant at first glance, but its contributions to the male reproductive system are monumental.

Location & Structure

Strategically positioned below the bladder, the prostate encircles the upper part of the urethra. Both ejaculatory ducts open within the urethra (the tube that urine and semen pass through) towards the back of the prostate. Semen flows from the seminal vesicles, through the ejaculatory ducts and then into the urethra.

The prostate sits directly in front of the rectum. The rectum is the lowest part of the intestines. This is where feces sit until it is ready to exit through the anus (Fig. 1). Because the rectum is so close to the prostate, when feces sits there and doesn't move, it can impact prostate health. During constipation, a ball of feces can sit directly behind the prostate, and through pressure and sometimes even the seepage of toxins from the feces through the thin wall that separates the two structures, it can impact the prostate.

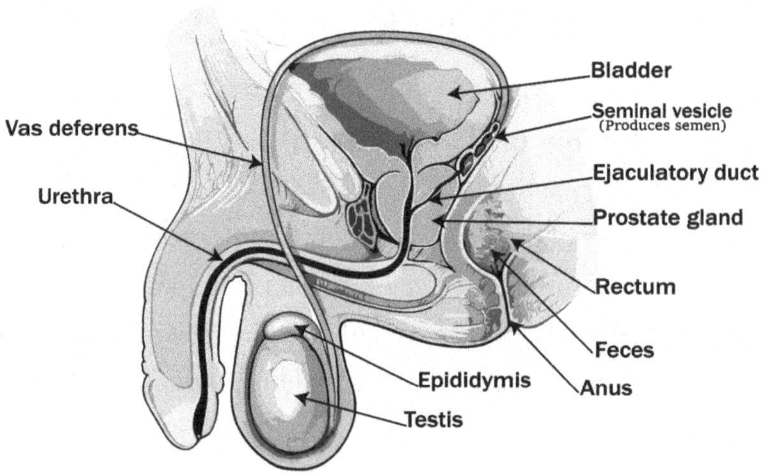

The prostate's location is actually purposeful. It serves as a crucial junction to both protect and produce. The prostate's muscular tissue aids in propelling seminal fluid (semen) into the urethra during ejaculation—comparable to the rubber band on a slingshot while the glands within the prostate produce vital fluid that actually supports and protects sperm.

The Prostate: The Unsung Hero of Reproduction

When most people think about reproduction, they mostly think of sperm. Those little swimmers are important because they hold the

DNA and the chromosomes of life. Without sperm, no pregnancies can occur. Imagine that sperm is present, but for some reason, it can no longer reach the intended target. Not because they have lost their ability to swim but because the river they intend to swim down is blocked off. This can happen when an enlarged prostate pushes into and narrows the tube that the sperm is intended to travel through: the urethra. This can also occur with prostatitis when the prostate is inflamed.

Or imagine the sperm is all lined up, ready to charge, and they cannot reach an egg to fertilize it because the prostate is weakened and cannot propel the sperm forward.

One of the primary functions of the prostate is the production of a thick, milky fluid, which constitutes about 30% of the total volume of semen. This fluid isn't just to make your load thicker. Prostatic fluid is a carrier. It protects the sperm and helps it get to an intended target. This thick fluid contains enzymes, sugar, citric acid, potassium, calcium, and fat. These nutrients provide essential nourishment for sperm cells that they require to swim safely to their intended destination. Think of prostatic fluid like the security detail for an important dignitary. Some leaders would never make it to their speeches alive without a security detail to drive and protect them on the way. Sperm, too, would be unhealthy and unable to swim without healthy prostatic fluid to escort and protect it along its way.

Additionally, prostatic fluid plays a role in neutralizing the acidity of the vaginal tract. The environment of the vagina is acidic. This thick fluid decreases the acidity of the vagina, ensuring that sperm cells can thrive and achieve fertilization.

Prostatic specific antigen (PSA) is released by the prostate into semen, and it actually waters the thick substance down so that the sperm are better able to move and swim. PSA can be elevated when inflammation is present when there is cancer present, when the prostate is enlarged, when chronic constipation is present, and even after sex.

Within the prostate, free testosterone is also converted to dihydrotestsoterone (DHT), which is a potent form of testosterone that is thought to encourage muscle formation, hair loss, and prostate growth.

Control Central: Erectile Function Nerve Hub

Yet another way that the prostate plays a role in fertility and reproduction is through the blood vessel-rich nerve structures that course both through and around the side of the prostate. The neurovascular bundle is a collection of nerves that runs along both sides of the prostate. In 2009, a study published in the European Journal of Urology[1] showed that when electrical stimulation is applied to the prostate between the 1 o'clock and the 5 o'clock position, they were able to create an erection. This proved that the network of nerves that surround the prostate contributes heavily

[1] https://pubmed.ncbi.nlm.nih.gov/18835086/

to the erectile process. You can see from Figure 2 how close these nerves are to the prostate and the rectum. Notice how the nerves travel all the way through to the corpus cavernosum of the penis, which is the muscular tissue of the erection.

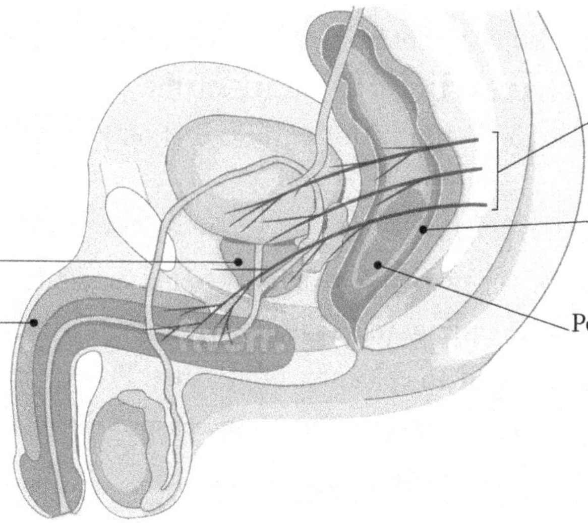

Once the network of nerves lodged within and surrounding the prostate becomes damaged either from the pressure of an enlarging prostate, inflammation, cancer, or surgery, this will interfere with erectile function. Without the ability to maintain an erection, of course, it will be more difficult to get someone pregnant.

Dual Functionality: Flow & Pleasure

Apart from its reproductive role, the prostate's muscular structure has another vital responsibility: it directs flow. The prostate acts as a switch, ensuring that urine and ejaculate don't mix. Have you ever wondered why you cannot pee and urinate at the same time? Well, during arousal, a complex interplay of nerves causes the prostate's muscles to contract, which blocks off the passageway from the bladder into the urethra. This ensures that only semen is propelled out during ejaculation.

Furthermore, the prostate's proximity to nerve bundles and its rich supply of nerve endings makes it a relay station for erectile function, but it also makes it an epicenter of pleasure. Proper prostate health isn't just about reproductive function; it's also intricately linked to the quality of male sexual experiences.

Guardian of Balance

The prostate serves as a soldier of balance. It helps maintain a delicate balance in the male reproductive system. It ensures the right pH for sperm, provides them with essential nutrients, and even aids in their transportation. Any malfunction or ailment affecting the prostate can throw this balance into disarray, affecting everything from reproductive health, sexual health, kidney function and general well-being.

The prostate also serves as a pathway for urine to exit from the bladder into the urethra and out into the world. If this pathway gets blocked or occluded, either through enlargement or with a mass, urine will back up into the bladder (Figure 3).

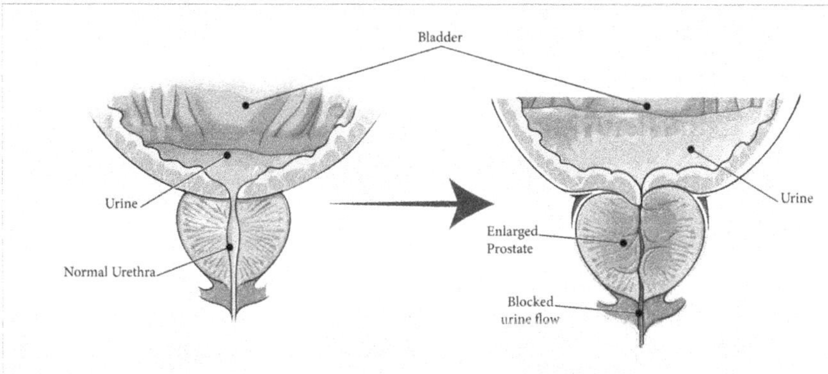

If urine cannot continuously flow freely through the prostate, the backup in the bladder will then cause the urine to back up into the kidneys, where urine is produced. Once this occurs, it can lead first to kidney disease through a process called hydronephrosis, and if it continues without relief, then kidney failure (Figure 4).

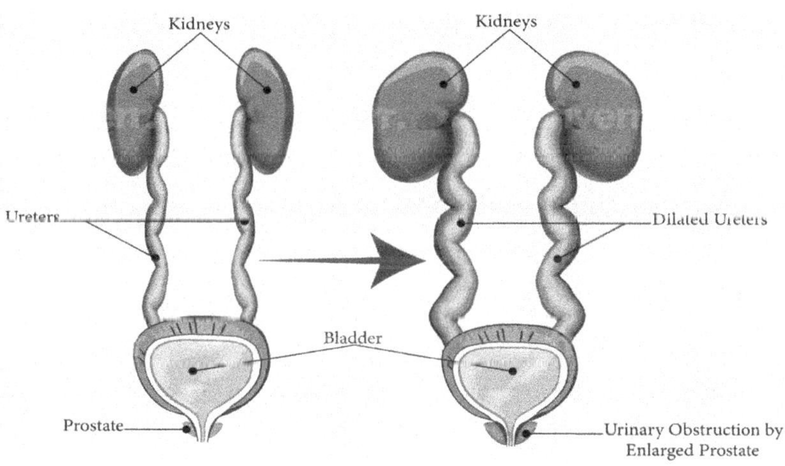

Once the prostate is enlarged (BPH), the silent backup of urine causes the bladder muscles to weaken or become what we call atonic. The need to rush to the bathroom every couple of hours increases and it can be a struggle to hold it. After urinating with an enlarged prostate, over time, there also may be some dribbling because the bladder wasn't emptied completely. For some, there is an urgent need to rush to the bathroom at night, which can interrupt the sleep cycle. An enlarged prostate wreaks havoc on the urinary tract. It can interfere with life, lifestyle, and intimacy.

In the grand scheme of male anatomy, the prostate is a silent workhorse, tirelessly performing its duties. Yet, it demands attention and care.

As we progress through this guide, the importance of nurturing this gland and recognizing its signals will become abundantly clear.

The Symbiotic Relationship

The relationship between the prostate and fertility is symbiotic. Just as the prostate influences fertility, factors affecting fertility (like infections, hormonal imbalances, or other conditions) can impact the prostate. It's a delicate balance, and understanding this interplay is essential for any man seeking to maintain or improve his reproductive health.

Prostate Health: The Key to Erection Quality

When discussing male sexual health, erections often take center stage. However, what many fail to recognize is the subtle yet pivotal role the prostate plays in influencing erection quality. The health of this small gland is intrinsically linked to a man's overall sexual well-being.

The Prostate-Erection Connection

To appreciate the connection, one must first understand the erection process. An erection is a complex dance of blood flow, neural signals, hormones, and muscular contractions. While the prostate doesn't directly cause erections, its health and functionality can significantly impact this intricate process.

1) Blood Flow: An ailing prostate, especially one swollen due to conditions like BPH, can impede the flow of blood in the pelvic region. Given that erections are fundamentally about blood flow to the penis, any restriction can impact erection quality and duration.

2) Neural Communication: The prostate is a nexus of nerve endings. Any inflammation or ailment affecting the prostate can interfere with the nerve signals essential for arousal and maintaining an erection.

3) Hormonal Balance: The prostate's health is closely tied to testosterone and dihydrotestosterone (DHT) levels. Any imbalance in these hormones, which play a key role in male sexual function, can indirectly affect erection quality.

The Ripple Effect of Prostate Conditions

Some men who experience prostate-related issues report challenges in multiple areas of their health:

- Pain and discomfort make arousal and maintaining an erection challenging
- Pain or discomfort during orgasm
- Urinary symptoms that indirectly affect a man's confidence and ability to maintain an erection
- Fertility issues
- Hesitant urine stream requiring a push to get the urine flow started
- Not making it to the bathroom (incontinence)
- Rushing to the bathroom (urgency)
- Constipation
- Getting up multiple times at night to urinate (nocturia)
- Decreased erectile stiffness (erectile dysfunction)
- Unable to ejaculate (anejaculation)
- Unable to orgasm (anorgasmia)
- Decreased volume of ejaculate
- Wet dreams

Prioritizing Prostate Health: A Step Towards Robust Erections

By taking proactive steps to maintain prostate health through regular check-ups, a balanced and healthy diet, exercise, and avoiding toxins as much as possible—one can bolster not only the prostate's well-being but also the overall quality of their sexual experiences. In essence, a healthy prostate can be a cornerstone for satisfying and robust erections.

Here are Some Useful Medical Terminology that You May Encounter:

- *Urinary retention* - leftover or retained urine in the bladder
- *LUTS (lower urinary tract symptoms)* - symptoms related to the bladder, prostate, and urethra
- *Cystoscopy* - a lighted tube that is about the size of a pencil is placed into the head of the penis to look inside the urethra and bladder and used to evaluate the size of the prostate.
- *Urinalysis or Urine dipstick*- a sample of urine is tested to detect infection, blood you cannot see, protein, and sugar in the urine.
- *Hematuria* - blood in the urine
- *Hydronephrosis* - urine backs up into the ureters (not to be confused with the urethra- see Figure 1 and Figure 4), which are tubes that usually carry urine away from the kidneys and into the bladder.
- *Urethral stricture* - a closed-down area of the urethra (compare it to a kink in a drinking straw)

- *Flow studies* - used to determine how much urine is coming out each time you urinate to help estimate how much stays stagnant in the bladder
- *Urodynamic studies* - used to see how the bladder fills and empties to see if the nerves are working properly
- *Overactive bladder (OAB)* - sudden and frequent urges to urinate that are hard to control
- *Incontinence* - urinating on yourself
- *Polyuria* - urinating 8 or more times a day or more than 2 times a night
- *Nocturia* - getting up more than once a night to urinate
- *Dysuria* - painful urination
- *Hematospermia* - blood in semen
- *STI testing - testing for infections you may have gotten while having sex.*
- *IPSS* - International prostate scoring symptom
- *Renal function testing* - blood tests to measure kidney function.
- *PSA* - prostatic specific antigen is a protein made by the tissue of the prostate- *prostate cancer can cause it to be elevated, but so can inflammation, constipation, exercise, sex*
- *DRE (digital rectal exam) - your healthcare provider places a gloved and lubricated finger into your rectum to feel the consistency and shape of the prostate.*
- *Prostate biopsy - tissue samples of the prostate are removed to be sent to the lab to inspect it underneath a microscope.*

CHAPTER 2:
THE SILENT EPIDEMIC: BENIGN PROSTATIC HYPERTROPHY

While the prostate might be small in size, the complications associated with it are anything but minor. For many men, prostate issues remain a silent affliction, manifesting subtly but escalating rapidly if left unaddressed. It's imperative to shed light on these conditions, not only for awareness but for proactive intervention.

Statistics: The Real Picture

In the quest to comprehend the scale and implications of prostate-related issues, numbers play an important role. It isn't just my dad or my loved ones with prostate-related issues. The numbers demonstrate the true magnitude of prostate disease.

How Many Men Will Have an Enlarged Prostate & When Will They Have It?

The Numbers: BPH (benign prostatic hypertrophy), or an enlarged prostate, affects a significant portion of the male population. It's estimated that over 50% of men in their 60s and as many as 90% in their 70s and 80s have some symptoms related to an enlarged prostate.

The Implication: As age increases, so does the likelihood of BPH.

Benign Prostatic Hyperplasia (BPH)

What is it? BPH is not cancer. It is an enlargement of the prostate gland. As the prostate enlarges, it can squeeze or block the urethra, leading to urinary symptoms.

Known Cause: Throughout the body, there is a balance that needs to be maintained. The cells are supposed to live and then die off. Within the prostate, when this balance is thrown off, and the rate of cells being produced outnumbers the cells that are dying, the prostate grows larger.

Suspected Contributors:

- Uncontrolled inflammation in the body
- Fake estrogens from environmental toxins
- Decreased testosterone but increased DHT
- Processed food
- Environmental hormone disruptors like food in plastics, food, clothing, home scents
- Exposure to phthalates, chemicals commonly found in soap, deodorant, fragrances, shampoos, and other personal care products, plastics, vinyl, and PVC products. Phthalates cause permanent harm to the male reproductive system, and they are so abundant

that this chemical has been named *the everywhere chemical* because it is literally everywhere. Phthalates are thought to increase BPH by disrupting hormone balance and tricking the body into increasing estradiol, DHT, and harmful reactive oxygen species.

- Oxidative stress

Risk Factors:

You are more likely to develop BPH if:

- You are obese, which is thought to make you have higher levels of inflammation and estrogen.
- You have diabetes or metabolic syndrome, which refers to a triad of conditions of prediabetes, high blood pressure, and high cholesterol.
- If you have a first-degree relative with BPH, you are four times more likely to develop BPH.
- If you are over the age of 50. 50% of men over the age of 50 are thought to have BPH.

The symptoms are the result of a combination of events. 1) obstruction comes from the size of the prostate compressing the urethra (think of a squeeze point in a straw that you are drinking) that causes a blockage as urine tries to leave the bladder. 2) the urine sits in the bladder because it becomes difficult to completely empty it all, and the bladder becomes irritated and weak. The symptoms associated with BPH are the result of prostate enlargement and the stagnant urine in the bladder.

When you have a fish tank or pond, you need the water to move and flow. If it doesn't flow, the stagnant water starts to grow bacteria, algae collects, and trouble ensues. Think of the bladder like the fish tank. It needs urine to flow. With stagnant urine, because the outlet is obstructed, instead of algae growing, bacteria will grow, and the muscle of the bladder gets weak or atonic.

Studies suggest that 75% of men with obstruction because of an enlarged prostate also have symptoms of overactive bladder (OAB). Overactive bladder is the frequent and uncontrollable urge to urinate.

Symptoms: Frequent urination, especially at night; difficulty starting or stopping a stream of urine; weak or interrupted urinary stream; a feeling of incomplete bladder emptying; painful bowel movements

Implications: Beyond the discomfort, BPH can lead to urinary tract infections, bladder stones, and kidney problems if untreated.

Common Complications:

- Urinary tract infections from urine sitting in the bladder too long
- Blood in the urine - as the prostate grows, blood vessels multiply, and the increased blood vessels can rupture and cause bleeding

- High pressure in the bladder from ongoing stagnant urine
- Kidney disease from the pressure building up in the bladder, which causes urine to back up into the kidneys
- Nighttime bed-wetting - high pressure of stagnant urine in the bladder seeps out at night

The Problem with BPH Meds

Navigating the world of medications for prostate health can feel like venturing into a dense forest. It's packed with potent solutions and hidden pitfalls that one should be wary of. Here's a closer look at some of the most frequently recommended medications and the potential side effects that aren't always at the forefront of discussions:

Alpha Blockers: Tamsulosin (Flomax), Terazosin, Doxazosin, Prazosin, Alfuzosin

How they work: Primarily prescribed to treat urinary symptoms due to an enlarged prostate or BPH (Benign Prostatic Hyperplasia). They function by relaxing the muscles in the prostate and the bladder neck, making it easier for urine to flow.

Hidden dangers: A benefit of alpha-blockers is that they start to work to mask symptoms almost right away. While effective at quickly minimizing some of the urinary symptoms associated with BPH, these drugs can come with side effects. Complaints of dizziness, headaches, nasal congestion, runny nose, and sometimes a significant drop in blood pressure. This sudden blood pressure drop can lead to fainting spells (orthostatic hypotension), particularly after the first dose. It's crucial to be aware and take precautions, especially if driving or operating heavy machinery.

Alpha-blockers can also cause retrograde ejaculation, which is ejaculate that shoots up into the bladder instead of out through the urethra. Alpha-blockers can also interfere with ejaculation, making it hard to do so, and it can lead to having little to no semen actually come out.

Caution When Taking the Blue Pill: They can cause sexual side effects, but you shouldn't take alpha-blockers with sildenafil or any of the other PDE-5 inhibitors like tadalafil, vardenafil, or avanafil. When taken together, there can be a dangerous and extreme drop in blood pressure.

Another more debilitating and perhaps the most common side effect is fatigue. Some users report feeling physically weak with a lack of energy and strength.

5-alpha reductase inhibitors:

Finasteride (Proscar, Propecia), Dutasteride (Avodart), Dutasteride/Tamsulosin (Jalyn)

How they work: These drugs block DHT. The most powerful form of testosterone. By doing so, the thought is that they can reduce the size and the symptoms of an enlarged prostate, offering relief from associated symptoms.

Hidden dangers: The FDA requires that these frequently prescribed drugs carry a warning label because they were shown clinically to increase the incidence of deadly forms of prostate cancer. Yes, you are reading that correctly. This drug is popularly used for male pattern hair loss because it blocks the production of DHT. But it can potentially contribute to a deadly form of prostate cancer. I am not even sure we should still be using these drugs.

Some men who take Finasteride can get persistent erectile dysfunction. In a study conducted at Northwestern University, men who took Dutasteride and Finasteride for longer periods of time had a higher risk of getting persistent erectile dysfunction. The erectile dysfunction in some of the men continued for months and, in some cases, years. The erectile dysfunction continued even after they stopped taking the meds. It even continued when they tried to take meds like Sildenafil (Viagra) to counteract the impact of the side effects.

The potential pitfalls here are multifaceted. Some men report a decrease in libido and a reduced volume of ejaculate. There's also an emotional and psychological dimension to consider.

5-alpha reductase inhibitors cross the barrier between the blood and the brain. Here, they block the production of certain nerve-related steroids. Blocked production can lead to struggles with mood swings, depression, and anxiety.

It is bad enough that there is an association with a variety of sexual side effects. Another potential issue is gynecomastia, which is an enlargement of breast tissue. Yes, on top of it all, some men grow boobs.

Antimuscarinics (oxybutynin, tolterodine):
BPH has related 'storage symptoms,' namely urgency to urinate and frequency of urination. Antimuscarinics were added with alpha-blockers to treat storage symptoms.

How they Work: These drugs block nerve signals that initiate the urination reflex. A recent meta-analysis study showed that adding these drugs doesn't seem to have any impact on the number of times a man rushes to the bathroom, and they appear to worsen and not improve retained urine.[2]

Hidden Dangers: There was a higher risk of acute urinary retention, which can be a medical emergency. Side effects included constipation and dry mouth.

---

[2] https://www.auajournals.org/doi/10.1097/JU.0000000000003077

Antispasmodics - Beta-3 Adrenergic Agonist (Myrbetriq, Mirabegron):

These drugs are medications designed to treat overactive bladder. An estimated 75% of men with BPH have clinical symptoms of an overactive bladder.[3] Beta-3 Adrenergic Agonists are the newest add-on for BPH patients with OAB. The suggested use in men with BPH is that they are to be taken with alpha-blockers to reduce urinary symptoms.

How they work: They work by relaxing the smooth muscle surrounding the bladder, allowing it to hold more urine. The bladder will spasm less, and the drug will delay the feeling that you need to empty your bladder.

Hidden Dangers: It can work too well and may cause urinary retention, making it too difficult to void. Myrbetriq should not be used in people with uncontrolled blood pressure as it can lead to a worsening in blood pressure. If there is obstruction of the outflow from the bladder. Also, in some people, a life-threatening swelling of the mouth and lips called angioedema may occur. Other side effects include urinary tract infection, constipation, abdominal pain, fatigue, and headache.

It may interact with blood thinners, some heart medications, antihistamines, antipsychotics, and some antidepressants.

---

[3] https://www.ncbi.nlm.nih.gov/pmc/articles/PMC3126063/#bibr14-1756287209350383

Prostate Meds: The Good, The Bad, & The Ugly

Beyond the direct, tangible side effects listed on the back of a pill bottle, there's a more insidious, often overlooked impact of medications on a man's overall sexual health and vitality. Here's a deeper exploration:

Diminished Sexual Desire: Medications, particularly those affecting hormonal balance, like 5-alpha reductase inhibitors, can have a profound effect on libido. Reduced interest in sexual activity can strain relationships, lead to feelings of inadequacy, and drastically alter one's quality of life. It's a subtle change, not always immediately attributed to medication, but it's real and concerning.

Erectile Dysfunction (ED): While ED can have multiple origins, certain prostate medications, especially those that interfere with hormone levels or blood flow, can either instigate or exacerbate the issue. ED doesn't only affect the physical act of intercourse but often brings along a host of emotional and psychological issues. The link between prostate meds and ED isn't always spelled out clearly to patients, and it's essential to be aware.

Ejaculatory Changes: Some men on prostate medications, particularly alpha-blockers, might notice changes in ejaculation. This could be a decreased volume of ejaculate or, in some cases, retrograde ejaculation, where the semen goes backward into the bladder instead of exiting the body.

Psychological Repercussions: The challenges of diminished libido, ED, and changes in ejaculation can lead to a cascade of psychological effects. Decreased self-confidence, anxiety, bouts of depression, and even identity crises can occur. Awareness of these potential emotional side effects is critical for the individual and their partners.

Recognizing and addressing the silent toll some medications can take on male sexual health and vitality is crucial. It's not about discarding these essential drugs but about understanding their full scope to make informed decisions and seek supportive interventions when necessary.

Why Are These Drugs So Readily Prescribed?

Medications play a central role in modern medicine. Their ability to alleviate symptoms, target specific physiological pathways, and improve quality of life is unparalleled. However, one can't help but wonder: Why are certain medications so quickly handed out, especially when they come with potential risks?

1) Dollars & Cents: Once a pharmaceutical company invests hundreds of millions of dollars into clinical trials, research and development, and marketing and then proceeds to bring it to market, the company's goal is to make money, period.

2) *Swift Symptom Relief*: Conditions like BPH can significantly hamper daily life, with symptoms like frequent urination, especially at night, or the inability to empty the bladder completely. Medications like alpha-blockers can provide rapid relief, restoring quality of life. The allure of quick symptom alleviation can often overshadow potential long-term side effects.

3) *Cost and Accessibility*: In many healthcare systems, medications are the most accessible and cost-effective intervention. Surgical procedures or other therapeutic options might be more invasive, expensive, or less readily available. In such scenarios, medication becomes the primary line of defense.

4) *Lack of Awareness or Discussion*: Sometimes, the potential side effects, especially those impacting sexual health, aren't discussed in depth. This might be due to a rushed consultation, the doctor's assumption that the patient is already informed, or an oversight into the significance of these side effects from a holistic well-being perspective.

5) *Pharmaceutical Influence*: While most doctors prioritize their patients' health, the pharmaceutical industry's influence can't be entirely discounted. Drug representatives, marketing campaigns, and financial incentives can, in some cases, sway prescription habits.

6) *Reliance on Band-Aid Syndrome:* These drugs mask the underlying cause of BPH, and, in many instances, they create a new set of problems for the person who relies heavily upon these things.

It's crucial to approach this topic with balance. On the one hand, medications are powerful tools in managing and mitigating prostate-related conditions, and their benefits can be life-changing. On the other hand, being an informed patient, asking questions, and weighing potential risks against benefits is vital. This proactive approach ensures that individuals receive care tailored to their unique needs and circumstances.

BPH

Procedures and Surgeries

Either because symptoms have not improved with medication or because the surgeon decides that surgery may be a better way to manage issues, some people opt for surgery—the promise that it will be like a miracle and 'quick and easy.' Some marketing terms used include 'minimally invasive,' 'in-office procedure,' and 'no downtime.'

The urologist often does not tell the patient that there may be disastrous complications. There may be pain, and their sex life may never be the same again.

A survey in the early 2000s found that 63% of urologists faced an average of 2 medical malpractice lawsuits.[4] Out of the procedures most associated with urologists being sued were TURP, transurethral resection of the prostate, 37%, transurethral microwave therapy, TUMT, 10%, and PVP, photovaporization of the prostate 10%.

Most of the time, these lawsuits are filed because afterward, the gent is not able to hold his urine anymore and instead must use adult diapers. Tied for the second most likely malpractice claim was the complaint of erectile dysfunction and urine retention.

It is a known fact that if the root cause of prostate enlargement is not addressed, the prostate will start to grow again after surgery. Although it is less clear in some of the newer procedures just how quickly this will happen, one in ten men will need a repeat procedure after having the most studied procedure, a TURP.

When deciding which surgical procedure to recommend, surgeons should consider the following:

- The size of the prostate
- Whether or not there is a large median lobe sticking out
- Whether or not the obstruction is caused by two lobes of the prostate being enlarged
- The cost of the procedure
- The physical condition of the patient

---

[4] https://www.ncbi.nlm.nih.gov/pmc/articles/PMC10284091/

Transurethral Resection of the Prostate (TURP):

TURP remains the standard surgical treatment for benign prostatic hyperplasia (BPH). This procedure is usually considered for men with moderate to severe urinary problems.

This is a 60 to 90-minute procedure, and it involves inserting an instrument called a resectoscope through the tip of the penis into the urethra and through to the prostate. The doctor does not have to make any cuts to your body for the procedure. Once it is within the prostate, the electrical loops from within the scope cut away the part of prostate tissue that is thought to be obstructing urine flow. It's typically performed under general or spinal anesthesia.

They typically keep you in the hospital for 1-2 days, and a catheter to drain urine is kept in place for up to 48 hours.

No sex for 4-6 weeks, and pain when you urinate may take 6-8 weeks to resolve.

Complications:

A recent prospective study examined data from 174 patients who had the TURP procedure. They found that 29.3% of these cases had some form of complication. Almost 10% had complications during surgery, 7.8% of them developed a urinary tract infection, 5.2% had perforated or hole poked into their prostate, stricture (closed off urethra) developed in 5.2%, and 4% of them needed to have a repeat operation. [5]

Short-term Complications: These include heavy bleeding, perforation of the capsule of the prostate, bladder injuries, urinary tract infection, infection, urinary retention, and TURP syndrome (a rare but potentially serious complication where the body absorbs too much fluid, leading to low sodium levels, confusion, and even seizures).

Long-term Complications: Some patients experience long-term effects such as strictures, retrograde ejaculation (semen flowing backward into the bladder), difficulty holding urine, erectile dysfunction, and urinary incontinence. Scar tissue formation can also occur, sometimes necessitating additional surgery. And potentially the need to retreat either because a stricture has returned or because it didn't work in the first place.

Cost: Typically between $5,000 to $15,000 in the United States, depending on the healthcare provider and insurance coverage.

UroLift® Procedure:

The UroLift® Procedure is designed to lift and hold the enlarged prostate tissue so it doesn't block the urethra. Think of it like tiny implants that stents open the pathway from the bladder through the urethra. It involves the placement of small implants that hold

---

[5] https://pubmed.ncbi.nlm.nih.gov/35813687/

the lobes of the prostate apart so that urine can flow. UroLift is performed under local or general anesthesia.

In a study that looked at complications between 2016 and 2023, the most common device problem was failure of the implant—which then required them to place a second one in position. Other complications included blood in urine, some of which required emergency surgery; five men had a stroke, and three had a pulmonary embolism; 22 people stayed in the hospital longer than 7 days, and eleven people died.[6] While the marketing materials

Things to keep in mind:

- It is less invasive than a TURP - but not as effective if you have a very large prostate and/or an enlargement of the median lobe of the prostate.
- It will not be effective if the person has a high bladder neck
- After putting you to sleep and putting you through a considerable process, the urologist actually will not have a tissue sample to send off to the lab to look for prostate cancer. With a TURP, there is tissue that can then be sent to the lab for analysis. A biopsy cannot be completed through this procedure.
- The implants can make MRI images hard to read later on if you need one.
- Some of the implants can become dislodged.
- The urologist doesn't know how many implants they are going to need when they go in. They charge per implant.

---

[6] https://journals.sagepub.com/doi/full/10.1177/03915603231180016

Expanded Complications:

Immediate Complications: Patients may experience discomfort during urination, bleeding, or pelvic pain shortly after the procedure.

Postoperative Concerns: In some cases, additional procedures might be needed if symptoms persist or if the implants displace.

Cost: Generally ranges from $8,000 to $14,600. Each implant will cost close to $1000 per implant, so it can be a costly procedure.

Rezūm Water Vapor Therapy:

Rezūm procedures are often performed on larger prostates that cannot be treated with the UroLift procedure. This procedure is usually completed in the office with local anesthesia. This therapy uses hot water vapor, or steam, to scald and destroy excess prostate tissue. The dead tissue is then left to be naturally reabsorbed by the body, and symptoms are supposed to decrease gradually over the course of two to three weeks.

Complications:

Immediate Postoperative Complications: Common risks include painful urination (16.9%), blood in the urine (11.8%), blood in semen (hematospermia), frequently rushing to the bathroom

(5.9%), urinary tract infections, or pelvic discomfort.[7] Discomfort following a Rezūm procedure usually lasts a few weeks. Most patients do not find immediate relief because the steam irritates the urinary tract.

Long-term Complications: Decreased ejaculatory volume. While it is less invasive, there's a potential for the regrowth of prostate tissue, leading to the return of symptoms over time. Also, some patients complain of urinary tract irritation for weeks following.
Cost: About $2,000 to $4,000, often covered by insurance

Transurethral microwave thermotherapy (TUMT)

Although rarely offered, TUMT is an option for men for whom surgery is not an option. It is usually performed in an outpatient setting, and numbness is usually achieved through a shot into your rectum or the area in between your scrotum and anus.

A small microwave antenna is then placed into the tip of the penis and inserted all the way to the prostate. A thermometer is placed into your anus to monitor the temperature so that it doesn't get too hot. Microwave energy is used to heat up and destroy the part of the prostate that is thought to be blocking the urine flow. The idea is that there is supposed to be just enough heat to damage a small amount of prostate tissue.

---

[7] https://pubmed.ncbi.nlm.nih.gov/30677455

Most men go home after the procedure with a urinary catheter in place to drain urine. With TUMT, it may take weeks or months to notice an improvement in symptoms.

Recently, the European Association of Urology withdrew its recommendation to use TUMT as a viable treatment option for BPH treatment. A disadvantage of the procedure is that the symptom improvement is short-lived. However, this is one of the few treatments that can actually be performed in an outpatient setting. One study found that 24% of the patients reported an improvement in erectile function after undergoing TUMT, which is something that most prostate surgical procedures cannot claim[8].

Short-term Complications: These include heavy bleeding, perforation of the capsule of the prostate, bladder injuries, urinary tract infection, infection, urinary retention, and TURP syndrome (a rare but potentially serious complication where the body absorbs too much fluid, leading to low sodium levels, confusion, and even seizures).

Long-term Complications: Some patients experience long-term effects such as strictures, retrograde ejaculation (semen flowing backward into the bladder), difficulty holding urine, erectile dysfunction, and urinary incontinence. Scar tissue formation can also occur, sometimes necessitating additional surgery. And potentially the need to retreat either because a stricture has returned or because it didn't work in the first place.

---

[8] https://www.ncbi.nlm.nih.gov/pmc/articles/PMC8276617/

Laser Enucleation & Laser Ablation: (HoLEP, HoLAP)

Once you are asleep, the surgeon inserts the resectoscope into your penis and up towards the prostate gland. Once in position, a laser is inserted into the resectoscope. Laser Enucleation (HoLEP—the ho is short for holium, which is a type of laser, and the LEP stands for laser enucleation of the prostate) usually uses a high-powered laser or photo-vaporization (greenlight laser) to enucleate (or remove part of it without cutting into it) the prostate.

The laser pulses beam into the prostate to cut out the overgrown tissue that is blocking the urine from flowing properly. They create a tunnel through the enlarged prostate so urine can flow through the part of the urethra within the prostate. Then, the laser is removed, and a morcellator is placed within the resectoscope. The prostate tissue that has been removed is chopped up and then sucked back out. The tissue is sent to the pathology department to be evaluated for cancer. The resectoscope is removed, and a catheter is placed within the urethra. The pros of this procedure are that it is designed to accomplish two things: both symptom relief and tissue biopsy (evaluation for cancer) at the same time.

Laser Ablation (HoLAP—the ho is short for holium, which is a type of laser, and the LEP stands for laser enucleation of the prostate) uses a high-powered laser or photo-vaporization to destroy the prostate tissue.

There are other types of high-powered lasers, and there will be even more as technology evolves. Please remember that a laser is only as good as the surgeon using it. A state-of-the-art laser with an untrained surgeon can have terrible outcomes.

Laser enucleation is not dependent on the size of the prostate. Even a very large prostate can be effectively treated using laser enucleation. Because they are actually removing tissue during this procedure.

Laser ablation is usually reserved for prostate size with volume <70-80mL.

The one caveat from laser surgery is that the physician usually doesn't tell you if he is planning to do laser enucleation or laser ablation. The decision is often made during the procedure. There is a huge difference. In an ablation, the tissue is destroyed or evaporated; in an enucleation, the tissue is retrieved.

The HoLEP removes more tissue than the HoLAP. On average, surgeons completing enucleation remove 50% to 60% of the prostate.

Laser procedures aim to provide relief from urinary symptoms while ideally preserving sexual function. But they require the skills of a highly trained surgeon. You want to ask your surgeon how many laser enucleation and/or ablation procedures they have performed. You also want to ask them how they personally determine which procedure will be done, enucleation versus ablation. Also, ask them which procedure they tend to perform more of and why.

Pay attention to your surgeon's body language. Are they annoyed with the line of questions, or are they comfortable answering? Are they giving you the pros and cons of all of your options?

Expect to have painful urination and to pee more frequently for the weeks that follow. Most surgeons will place you on an anti-inflammatory medication and a medication to ease bladder spasms. You also may have to wear pads in your underwear for a few days as it may be difficult to control your urine.

Procedure-specific Risks:

Most people can return to work within 2 weeks unless the job is strenuous. Laser procedures are thought to reduce the risk of bleeding (so they are better for patients who have a bleeding risk), the need to repeat the procedure, and decrease the need for an overnight hospital stay.

Less than 2% of people who undergo laser enucleation require a second surgery.

Anytime someone is put to sleep for surgery, there is a risk of blood clots, heart attacks, or aspiration. With laser surgery, there is a risk of injury to the urethra, the bladder, and the ureters.

Short-term Risks: May include catheter-related discomfort, urinary urgency, bleeding when you pee, infection, excessive bleeding, or need for temporary self-catheterization.

Long-term Risks: 75% will no longer be able to ejaculate. Possible long-term risks include urinary incontinence and erectile dysfunction if nerves are injured in the process.

Cost: Typically ranges from $6,000 to $20,000

Ablation Therapy:

Ablation is a generalized term for vaporizing or destroying the prostate tissue. Radiofrequency or cryo ablation therapy destroys prostate tissue by applying extreme temperatures. Cryoablation freezes the tissue, while radiofrequency ablation uses high-frequency energy to heat and destroy cells.

Expanded Risks:

Procedure-specific Risks: Cryoablation carries a risk of tissue sloughing, where dead cells may obstruct the urethra, while radiofrequency ablation can sometimes lead to more extensive damage due to heat.

General Risks: These include a risk of erectile dysfunction and urinary incontinence, as well as the potential for injury to the rectum, given the prostate's proximity.

Cost: Can be upwards of $15,000, with prices varying widely.

Economic and Personal Impact

The cost of prostate surgical procedures can be significant, with variations depending on geographic location, facility, insurance, and the specific needs of the patient. It's not just the immediate financial burden that's concerning; indirect costs such as time off work, recovery, and potential complications can lead to further medical expenses.

These procedures carry risks, and they should not be taken lightly. The term minimally invasive can sometimes be misleading. So, ask questions, do your homework, and by all means, try to keep your prostate as healthy as possible so that maybe you can avoid needing prostate surgery.

The Case for Natural Prostate Management

By focusing on a natural approach to prostate health, some men will be able to avoid these procedures. A dedicated routine involving diet, exercise, and possibly supplements may support prostate function and mitigate symptoms associated with BPH. However, it is vital to understand that while a natural approach can be highly effective for some, it is not a guarantee against prostate disease, and regular medical consultation remains essential.

CHAPTER 3:
PROSTATITIS

Prostatitis is the most common urinary issue in men who haven't yet had their fiftieth birthday. It is not a cancer and having it does not appear to increase your risk of developing prostate cancer. Prostatitis refers to inflammation or swelling of the prostate gland. It can be acute (short-term) or chronic (long-term) and might be due to infections or other non-infectious factors. Prostatitis, for many men, is extremely painful.

Risk Factors:

- Prostatitis is more common in middle-aged men
- An infection transmitted sexually
- Injury to the pelvis
- A recent infection of the urinary tract
- Having had a prostate biopsy
- A catheter has recently been placed to drain urine from the bladder
- Having received anal sex recently

Symptoms: Pain or discomfort in the groin, painful ejaculation, pain in the penis, pain in the testicles, pain in the area between the testicles and the anus, running to the bathroom frequently, blood in semen; painful ejaculation, problems with erections; and flu-like symptoms in the case of acute bacterial prostatitis.

Suspected Contributors:

- **Inflammation:** Chronic inflammation within the prostate or surrounding tissues can lead to nerve irritation or damage. Inflammatory cells can release substances that affect nerve function and cause pain.
- **Trauma:** Direct trauma to the pelvic region, such as an injury or following surgery.
- **Physical Stress:** Repetitive activities or strain, including activities like cycling or heavy lifting, can put pressure on the pelvic nerves and the prostate and lead to inflammation.
- **Bladder infections**
- **Autoimmune Reactions:** Some cases of prostatitis may involve autoimmune reactions, where the body's immune system mistakenly attacks healthy prostate cells and nerves, causing chronic pain and inflammation.
- **Neurological Disorders:** Underlying neurological conditions that affect nerve health can also contribute to the development of chronic prostatitis symptoms.
- **Psychological Factors:** Stress and anxiety can lead to muscle tension in the pelvic floor, which can put pressure on nerves and lead to pain. This is often addressed with therapies that focus on relaxing the pelvic floor muscles.
- **Hormonal Imbalances:** Hormones play a role in regulating inflammation and nerve

health. Imbalances, particularly of testosterone and estrogen, may contribute to sensitivity and inflammation around the pelvic nerves.

Potential Complications

A person can become septic if prostatitis has been caused by bacteria, resulting in a shutdown of the organ systems.

Implications: Chronic prostatitis can significantly affect quality of life, leading to persistent pain and discomfort, sexual dysfunction, and psychological distress.

Prevention of Prostatitis:

Drink Lots of Water:

This can help flush bacteria from the bladder and urinary tract.

Urinate Regularly:

Avoid holding urine for long periods, as this can increase the risk of bacterial infection.

Use Condoms:

Reduce the risk of STIs, which can lead to prostatitis, by using condoms and engaging in safe sex practices.

Avoid Activities that Irritate the Prostate:

Activities such as cycling, or horseback riding can irritate the prostate; using a padded seat or taking frequent breaks can help.

Manage Stress:

Chronic stress can lead to symptom flare-ups. Manage stress through techniques like meditation, exercise, or therapy.

Diet:

Avoid or limit caffeine, alcohol, and spicy foods, which can irritate the prostate.

Pelvic Floor Exercises:

Strengthening pelvic floor muscles can help in managing chronic prostatitis symptoms.

Regular STI Checks:

Get tested for sexually transmitted infections regularly.

Warm Baths:

For those with prostatitis, warm baths can help soothe pain and inflammation.

Therapeutic Massage:

Some individuals find relief from chronic prostatitis symptoms with prostate massage, which can reduce inflammation and alleviate pain. There is published data on using a combination of antibiotics with prostate massage in order to treat chronic prostatitis. However, massage should not be performed during a flare-up.

CHAPTER 4:
THE OVERDONE & OVERSOLD PROSTATE BIOPSY

The Overdone Prostate Biopsy:

More than 1 million prostate biopsies are completed each year. When the doctor suggests that a prostate biopsy be done, it is a natural knee-jerk reaction to mistrust the suggestion. I think urologists who perform the procedure do them so often that they have convinced themselves that they are really no big deal. If they are done in-office and without any complications, the average cost of a prostate biopsy is $1750[9]. So, it is easy to see why they are performed so often. An estimated 75% of prostate biopsies are found not to be cancerous. That means that 75% of men who have undergone a prostate biopsy really didn't need one.

Common Prostate Biopsy Complications:

1) **Bleeding:** Some bleeding is common after a prostate biopsy. You might notice blood in your urine or semen, which usually isn't cause for concern and should clear up within a few weeks. Rectal bleeding is also possible but typically light and short-lived.

[9] https://pubmed.ncbi.nlm.nih.gov/37317377/

2) **Infection:** There's a small risk of infection after a biopsy. The risk is reduced by taking antibiotics before and after the procedure as prescribed by your doctor. If you experience fever, chills, or severe pain, it's important to contact your healthcare provider immediately, as these may be signs of an infection.

3) **Pain and Discomfort:** It's normal to experience pain or discomfort in the area where the biopsy was taken. Pain relief medication can help manage this.

4) **Difficulty Urinating:** Some men might find it difficult to urinate following the procedure. This is usually temporary, but if you're unable to urinate for several hours or if there's significant pain, you should seek medical attention.

5) **Erectile Dysfunction:** While it is a less common side effect, some men may experience erectile dysfunction (ED) following a prostate biopsy. This is generally temporary and should resolve without treatment.

Less Common Complications:

- **Prostatitis:** Inflammation of the prostate gland (prostatitis) can occur, which may require treatment with antibiotics.

- **Urinary Retention:** In rare cases, swelling caused by the biopsy can block urine flow, requiring temporary catheterization.

Severe Complications:

Severe complications from prostate biopsies are rare but can include:

- **Sepsis:** This is a potentially life-threatening condition that occurs when an infection spreads throughout the body. Immediate medical treatment is crucial.
- **Hospitalization:** While the risk is low, hospitalization may be needed if severe infection or bleeding occurs.

My frustration with an unnecessary prostate biopsy is that it can actually damage the lives of men. The surgeon goes home and makes money for his group, while the patient heads home with worsened symptoms because the surgeon blindly proceeds to conduct a 12-needle biopsy. 12 needles are placed randomly within the prostate tissue. This is like saying, 'we think we have a cancer, so we are just going to randomly stick 12 needles into your prostate and see what we find.' It is pretty absurd if you think about it.

Then this same surgeon may get the pathology results back and then overtreat what he thinks is an aggressive prostate cancer, which may not have been, and now the patient unnecessarily has leaking urine, ED, a stressed existence, or maybe all of the above.

Unfortunately, this happens to hundreds of thousands of men each year. Some doctors see an elevated PSA and immediately decide to biopsy and treat it. This is overtreating and over diagnosing prostate cancer.

Timing and Frequency of Prostate Biopsy as per AUA Guidelines:

According to the AUA, the decision to perform a prostate biopsy should be individualized, taking into account each man's unique clinical situation, including PSA levels, physical exam findings, and personal risk factors. The AUA emphasizes the importance of shared decision-making between the patient and the healthcare provider, ensuring that the decision to proceed with a biopsy is made with a full understanding of the potential benefits and risks involved.

Initial Biopsy: Should be considered based on a combination of PSA levels, DRE results, patient age, comorbidities, and patient preference.

Repeat Biopsy: This may be indicated if PSA levels rise or if a patient has a negative initial biopsy but continues to have clinical signs suggestive of prostate cancer.

Surveillance Biopsy: The frequency of surveillance biopsies can vary; the AUA suggests a discussion between the patient and healthcare provider to decide on appropriate intervals.

I believe there are three ways that biopsies could and should be handled in order to decrease the number of unnecessary ones.

1) After an elevated PSA level, get a multiparametric MRI. This type of MRI scan produces a detailed picture of the prostate gland. If the MRI shows suspicious areas, then do a biopsy. A recent study conducted in Sweden made it clear that if surgeons find elevations in the PSA and then order an MRI of the prostate to look for suspicious areas of the prostate and subsequently only biopsied any suspicious areas, they could essentially reduce the risk of over-biopsying and over-diagnosing prostate cancer by 50%.[10] This huge study invited over 37,000 men 50-60 years of age to get a PSA level. If their PSA was 3ng or more, they were assigned to certain treatment groups.

The problem with this approach is that the average charge for a prostate MRI is $4,419.[11] Most insurance companies will find a way to avoid paying for this test.

2) After an elevated PSA test, an exosome test could be done. The exosome prostate test uses your urine sample to analyze and look for exosomes that hold information on prostate cancer-specific biomarkers.

[10] https://pubmed.ncbi.nlm.nih.gov/36177032/

[11] https://healthimaging.com/topics/medical-imaging/magnetic-resonance-imaging-mri/prostate-mri-pricing-among-us-facilities

The biomarkers are measured, and then they use an algorithm to calculate a score to determine the risk that the man has clinically significant or aggressive prostate cancer. It is designed to be used for men over 50 with PSA levels ranging from 2 - 10ng/mL. If the ExoDX intelliscore is >15.6, this means there is a higher risk that an aggressive or clinically significant cancer is present.

After the results are in, the patient and the physician can make an informed choice to proceed to MRI and potentially move on to biopsy. The test allows you to work with your physician to make a decision based on your own personal risk. The ExoDx Prostate test can be completed at home. At the time of this publication, it had been proven to avoid almost 30% of biopsies.

The ExoDX Prostate Test has a negative predictive value (NPV) of 91%, which means that the results will show with 91% certainty that the person will not have an aggressive form of prostate cancer if the score is 15.6 or less.

3) Ultimately, combining a multiparametric prostate MRI with a test like the exosome ExoDX Prostate test may even be the most complete option. It is time that prostate cancer evaluation takes on a personalized approach. That way, patients can adequately weigh the benefits and the risks before an invasive prostate biopsy is done.

So much of the fear and hesitation towards prostate biopsy comes from the fact that patients know it may be a waste of their time and that it is not as simple of a procedure as they have made it out to be.

The exosome prostate test costs about $150 out of pocket.

Questions to ask your doctor once they recommend you have a prostate biopsy:

What is my PSA level, and how have my PSA levels changed over time?

How accurate is the PSA in assessing my risk for high-grade prostate cancer?

What is the chance of having a negative or undetermined result for prostate cancer if I have a prostate biopsy?

What is the treatment plan if my prostate biopsy results in a "Low Grade" prostate cancer?

What are alternatives to a prostate biopsy for diagnosis of prostate cancer?

Is there any risk to obtaining The ExoDx Prostate Test before the biopsy?

Can I get an MRI of the prostate before we settle on doing a biopsy at this time?

What do you think will happen if I don't get a prostate biopsy right now?

The Role of MRI in Assessing Prostate Health Before a Biopsy

When you're navigating the uncertain waters of prostate health, an MRI scan can be a valuable tool before considering a biopsy. MRI stands for Magnetic Resonance Imaging, and it uses a powerful magnetic field, radio waves, and a computer to produce detailed pictures of the inside of your body.

What is an MRI for Prostate Health?

An MRI of the prostate provides a clear image of the prostate gland and the surrounding tissue. Unlike a PSA test, which gives an indirect indication of a problem through the measurement of proteins in the blood, an MRI provides a direct look at the prostate. This can be incredibly helpful for doctors to see if any areas look unusual and might need a closer check with a biopsy.

Why Get an MRI Before a Biopsy?

An MRI can sometimes find cancers that a PSA test might miss, and it can also help to avoid unnecessary biopsies. Here's why an MRI is an important consideration before a biopsy:

Targeted Imaging: MRI scans can show more detailed images, which can help locate specific areas within the prostate that may need to be sampled during a biopsy.

Minimizing Risk: By providing a clearer picture, an MRI can reduce the chances of going through an unnecessary biopsy, which can have side effects and risks.

Guiding Biopsies: If a biopsy is needed, an MRI can help guide the procedure to ensure that the right area of the prostate is sampled.

Monitoring: For men under "active surveillance" for prostate cancer, MRIs can be used to monitor the prostate over time without needing multiple biopsies.

The MRI Process

Getting an MRI scan usually follows these steps:

Consultation: Your doctor will evaluate if an MRI is appropriate for you based on your PSA levels, physical exam, and medical history.

The Scan: You'll be asked to lie down on a table that slides into the MRI machine, which is a long tube that's open at both ends. The machine is loud, but you'll often be given earplugs or headphones.

Duration: An MRI scan can take from 30 minutes to an hour. During this time, you'll need to stay still to get clear images.

Contrast Agent: Sometimes, a contrast material might be used to enhance the visibility of certain structures in the image.

After the Scan: You can usually return to normal activities after an MRI.

Understanding the ExoDx Prostate Test: A Non-Invasive Game Changer

Navigating the uncertainties of prostate health can be daunting, especially when it comes to distinguishing between benign conditions and prostate cancer. The ExoDx Prostate (IntelliScore), or EPI, is a cutting-edge, non-invasive urine test that is changing the game in prostate health management. Here's what you need to know:

Every year, doctors complete about 500,000 biopsies to look for cancer. But sometimes, these checks may not be needed. When someone has prostate cancer, the way it shows up can be different for each person. Knowing what kind of prostate cancer is helps doctors figure out the best way to treat it and what problems they might run into.

1. What is the ExoDx Prostate Test?

The ExoDx Prostate Test is a genomic urine test that helps in assessing the risk of high-grade prostate cancer. It measures the levels of three specific RNA biomarkers associated with aggressive prostate cancer.

2. How Does It Work?

The test analyzes the genetic material from exosomes, which are tiny vesicles released from cells, including cancer cells, found in urine. By measuring these biomarkers, the test generates an EPI score that indicates the likelihood of high-grade prostate cancer on a scale from 0 to 100.

3. Who Should Take This Test?

The test is designed for men who are 50 years and older with a PSA level of 2-10 ng/mL and who have not had a previous prostate biopsy.

4. Benefits of the ExoDx Prostate Test

The test only requires that you urinate in a special collection cup. The test can be performed at home or in your doctor's office.

5. How to Get the Test

Your doctor can order the test and provide you with a collection kit, or you can order a test online through the ExoDx website. Once you provide your urine sample, you mail it off, and the results are typically available to your doctor within a few days.

6. The Results

The results are all about risk stratification. The whole purpose of this test is to help you and your physician use an educated risk analysis to determine whether or not you should proceed with a biopsy at this time.

If You Still Aren't Sure, Get a Second Opinion:

When you're faced with the prospect of a prostate biopsy, and you are feeling uneasy about it, it's crucial to ensure that the decision is sound. One of the best ways to feel confident in your healthcare choices is to seek a second opinion from a urologist outside of the clinic group. Here's why:

Confirmation of Diagnosis:

A second opinion can confirm whether the initial diagnosis and biopsy recommendation are consistent with another healthcare professional's findings.

Expertise and Experience:

Doctors have different levels of expertise and experience with prostate health, so they may have different opinions. A second doctor might suggest alternative tests or monitoring approaches that could delay or even eliminate the need for a biopsy. They might also provide a different interpretation of test results, such as PSA levels, potentially leading to a different course of action.

Peace of Mind:

Knowing that two independent medical professionals agree on a course of action can provide significant peace of mind. It also ensures that you are more informed about your condition and the necessity of a biopsy.

Additional Options:

A second opinion might reveal additional treatment or monitoring options you were unaware of.

Insurance Considerations:

Some insurance plans cover second opinions for serious conditions like potential prostate cancer. Some plans even require a second opinion before certain procedures, so it's wise to check your policy.

How to Get a Second Opinion:

Ask around. Ask family and friends that you know have had prostate procedures in the past. Look online, read reviews and look for medical centers specializing in holistic prostate care or functional medicine. These clinics typically take a more conservative approach to prostate care. Most of these clinics will offer you an online consultation, and you can get an informative consultation without the need to travel.

Prostate Biopsy - What to Expect

It is important to take prostate biopsy seriously. Take the time to make sure you really need one.

The two most common types of prostate biopsy are the transrectal and the transperineal prostate biopsies. The transrectal biopsy involves a needle passing through the wall of the rectum to perform the biopsy. In the second method, a needle is inserted through the area of skin between the anus and the scrotum; this is the transperineal prostate biopsy.

The transrectal biopsy has a higher infection and complication rate because the needle passes through the rectal wall in order to retrieve the biopsy sample.

Transperineal biopsies are the gold standard, and they are considered clean because the needle goes through the perineum, not the rectum. The transperineal approach decreases the rate of infection from 40 to 70%. The biopsy can be performed under local anesthetic, where they numb the area by injecting a numbing agent around the pudendal nerve, or they can put you to sleep.

Then, an ultrasound probe is placed into your rectum to help visualize the prostate and help your physician decide where to take the biopsies from. The surgeon proceeds to use the needle to poke 12-15 holes into the prostate. Each needle punch is a biopsy, and the tissue is sent to the lab for analysis.

Potential complications of prostate biopsy might include infection, bleeding, bruising, pain, trouble urinating, and blood in urine or semen.

CHAPTER 5: PROSTATE CANCER

The whole purpose of a prostate biopsy is to uncover and detect prostate cancer. Prostate cancer is tricky. A normal PSA level doesn't necessarily mean you don't have prostate cancer, as 15% of men with normal PSA levels can still have prostate cancer.[12] And 75% of men with elevated PSA levels end up not having prostate cancer. So, there still really isn't an adequate screening tool for prostate cancer.

I am old-school, and I believe that all men should have a digital rectal exam (DRE) each year. If your trained healthcare provider places their finger on your prostate, he or she can feel abnormalities on the surface of the gland, but it will not allow for the detection of any tumors deep within the gland.

Once PSA levels reach 4ng/mL, it is considered 'suspicious.' I always repeat any elevated PSA because so many things can cause it to be elevated. Once we are sure that the PSA is, in fact, elevated, the hard work comes next. As a family physician, my goal is to always work with my patients to be a liaison and a gatekeeper between the patient and the specialist. Surgeons can make decisions to operate

[12] https://pubmed.ncbi.nlm.nih.gov/15163773/

based on a variety of things like money, their golf schedule, timing, and sometimes even quota numbers. My job has always been to make sure that the decision to biopsy or treat aligns with what my patient needs and wants.

Global and Regional Prostate Cancer Statistics: Incidence, Mortality, and Survival Rates

The Numbers: Prostate cancer stands as the second most common cancer in men worldwide. The World Health Organization (WHO) notes that over 1.4 million cases of prostate cancer were diagnosed in 2020 alone.

The Implication: The prevalence of prostate cancer remains a global concern.

The Reality of Prostate Cancer and BPH: What the Numbers Say

The Numbers: While BPH and prostate cancer are distinct conditions, their symptoms often overlap. It's estimated that about 10-12% of men with BPH symptoms eventually get diagnosed with prostate cancer. However, it's crucial to note that BPH does not increase the risk of prostate cancer, nor does it seem to cause it.

The Implication: The overlap in symptoms emphasizes the importance of symptom management. Men with urinary symptoms should not dismiss them as 'just BPH' but should seek medical evaluation to rule out malignancies.

Prostate cancer is a malignant growth within the prostate. While many prostate cancers grow slowly, some can be aggressive, making early detection crucial.

If you are Black and/or have a family history of prostate cancer, you should speak with your doctor at 40 about screening. But you should start putting a healthy prostate plan together before that.

Symptoms: Early-stage prostate cancer often has no symptoms. As it progresses, one might experience urinary symptoms, blood in semen, erectile dysfunction, pain in the hips or back, or unexplained weight loss.

Implications: Prostate cancer is among the leading causes of cancer deaths in men. Early detection and appropriate treatment can significantly increase the chances of survival.

Risk Factors:

- Older age
- Family history
- Being Black - 1 in 6 Black men will be diagnosed with prostate cancer. Black men are almost 2 times as likely to be diagnosed with prostate cancer and 2 times more likely to die of prostate cancer than white men.
- Genetics
- Agent Orange exposure during the Vietnam War
- Obesity

Prevention & Early Detection

You know yourself better than anyone. You know your body, and when something doesn't feel right. And when it doesn't, you must go to the doctor to get evaluated.

If you have a family history of prostate cancer or a personal history of chronic disease, you are at an increased risk of developing prostate cancer.

Prostate Cancer: Recognizing the Warning Signs

Often, prostate cancer can progress without noticeable symptoms, making vigilance and regular screenings crucial. However, there are signs that should prompt immediate medical consultation:

1) **Urinary Changes:** Difficulty starting urination, a weak or interrupted flow, the need to urinate more frequently, especially at night, or an inability to empty the bladder fully can be early signs of prostate cancer.

2) **Blood Presence:** The appearance of blood in urine or semen is a stark indicator that something is amiss and warrants immediate medical attention.

3) **Pain or Discomfort:** Persistent pain in the lower back, hips, thighs, or pelvic area can be a sign of advanced prostate cancer, which may have spread to the bones.

4) **Erectile Dysfunction:** Difficulty achieving or maintaining an erection can be an early sign of prostate cancer and should be evaluated in the context of other symptoms.

5) **Weight Loss:** Unexplained weight loss is a nonspecific symptom but can be associated with advanced cancer.

6) **Back Pain:** Prostate cancer can spread to the bones, and back pain can be a sign of cancerous growth in the spine.

These are the more overt signs, but there are subtler ones that should not be ignored:

1) **Subtle Discomfort:** A mild, often overlooked discomfort or pressure in the pelvic area, which might be mistaken for something benign, can be an early warning sign.

2) **Changes in Ejaculation:** Pain or discomfort during ejaculation, or a noticeable decrease in the amount of seminal fluid, could suggest prostate issues.

3) **Leg Swelling or Weakness:** In rare cases, prostate cancer may cause swelling in the legs or feet or cause weakness in the legs.

4) **Constipation:** The prostate gland is situated below the bladder, encircling the urethra, and is in close proximity to the rectum. An enlarged prostate due to cancer can press on the rectum, leading to constipation.

What Causes Prostate Cancer?

People assume that BPH is likely to turn into prostate cancer, but this is not true. It is quite the opposite. Recent studies indicate that the larger one's prostate actually is, the less likely it is that he will develop prostate cancer.[13] A large prostate actually appears to be protective against deadly forms of prostate cancer.

Most prostate cancer starts in the part of the prostate known as the peripheral zone, and BPH is usually localized within the inner or transitional zone of the prostate. Enlarged prostates are actually less likely to develop deadly forms of prostate cancer.[14] This may explain the fact that highly prescribed prostate medications like Finasteride and Dutasteride (Proscar, Propecia, AVodart) are required to put a warning on the box that this class of drugs, known as 5-alpha reductase inhibitors, may be linked to an increased risk of developing an aggressive form of prostate cancer.

Prostate cancer is the second most common cancer among men, and theories abound about the cause, but two factors increasingly scrutinized are the toxins we see around us, xenobiotics and estrogens.

Xenobiotics: These are foreign chemical substances that are completely foreign to our bodies. These include a wide range of chemicals, from pesticides to cosmetics to flavorings and industrial

---

[13] https://www.beaumont.org/health-wellness/press-releases/researchers-enlarged-prostate-lowers-odds-of-significant-prostate-cancer

[14] https://dx.doi.org/10.14218/ERHM.2022.00120

agents. They are suspected of playing a huge role in the onset of prostate cancer. Some xenobiotics alter your DNA, some enter the body and act like estrogen, some block hormonal actions, some trigger immune responses within the body, and some do all of the above. The concern is that these substances can potentially alter hormone systems within the body, leading to altered prostate cells and, over time, creating an environment where cancerous cells could thrive.

Estrogens: There's a growing body of research exploring how estrogens—and their interaction with other hormones like testosterone—may influence prostate cancer risk. While estrogens are crucial hormones even in the male body, an imbalance, particularly an excess, may contribute to prostate cancer. Estrogens can build up in the tissue of the prostate and also throughout the body. When your body attempts to remove some of it, it can stay stuck in the body and increase the number of cancer cells.

Estrogen in the environment builds up. Humans push estrogen out into urine and feces, as do the animals we eat. It's in the fertilizers; the animals we eat are given estrogen, and estrogens are in large amounts in our water supply.

Estrogen and estrogen-like compounds are everywhere.

Our Great Lakes have so much estrogen in them that even fish populations are becoming feminized.

Xenoestrogens and estrogen appear to be fueling prostate disease. But they also limit fertility. Fertility is limited even further after prostate cancer treatment. After treatment, there is a reduced ability to conceive naturally. The potential fertility impacts of environmental estrogens and other endocrine disruptors, while still being understood, hint at a broader reproductive crisis.

Prostate cancer is a multifaceted disease with various potential causes and risk factors. Beyond xenobiotics and estrogen exposure, here are other recognized contributors to the development of prostate cancer:

Genetic Factors: A family history of prostate cancer can increase a man's risk. Specific gene mutations or SNPs that can now be easily tested for are also known to elevate the risk.

Age: The risk of prostate cancer increases with age, particularly after the age of 50. It's most common in men over 65.

Race and Ethnicity: African American men have a higher incidence of prostate cancer and are more likely to die from the disease than men of other races. The reasons for this are complex.

Diet and Lifestyle: A diet high in red meat, high-fat dairy products, and low in fruits and vegetables may increase the risk. Obesity is also associated with an elevated risk of aggressive prostate cancer.

Hormonal Influences: High levels of androgens, such as testosterone, have been associated with prostate cancer risk. The prostate is an androgen-sensitive organ, and while androgens do not cause prostate cancer per se, they are necessary for prostate cancer to develop.

Inflammation: Chronic inflammation of the prostate, which could be due to a variety of reasons, including sexually transmitted infections, may increase the risk of developing prostate cancer.

Sexual Factors: There is some evidence to suggest that a history of sexually transmitted infections (STIs) may be linked to an increased risk of prostate cancer due to chronic inflammation.

Environmental Exposure: Occupational exposure to certain chemicals, like those used in farming and metalworking, may increase prostate cancer risk.

Lifestyle Factors: Lack of exercise and a sedentary lifestyle have been linked to an increased risk of prostate cancer.

Geographical Factors: Prostate cancer is more common in North America and northwestern Europe, suggesting that environmental factors like diet, lifestyle, and medical practices may play a role.

Vitamin and Mineral Deficiencies: Some studies suggest that low levels of vitamin D and certain minerals might be linked to an increased risk of prostate cancer, although the evidence is not definitive.

Understanding these factors is essential in developing a comprehensive prevention strategy. It's important to note that having one or more risk factors does not mean a man will get prostate cancer, and many men with the disease may not have any apparent risk factors.

This complex interplay of genetic, environmental, and lifestyle factors underscores the need for personalized approaches to prostate cancer prevention, screening, and treatment. It also highlights the importance of ongoing research to unravel the intricate mechanisms behind the initiation and progression of prostate cancer.

Prostate Cancer: Reduce Your Risk

Dietary Choices

- Eat more fruits and vegetables: These foods are rich in vitamins and antioxidants, which can protect the cells in your body.
- Choose whole-grain foods over refined grains.
- Reduce intake of red meat that is not organic, antibiotic-free, or hormone-free. Instead, make sure your red meat is grass-fed and as organic as possible. Limit processed meats. Eating more red meat and processed meat may be associated with an increased risk of prostate cancer.[15]

---

[15] https://www.ncbi.nlm.nih.gov/pmc/articles/PMC8859108/

Maintain a Healthy Weight:

- Obesity has been linked with an increased risk of dying from prostate cancer.[16] Working towards a healthy weight through diet and exercise could help lower the risk.

Exercise Regularly:

- Physical activity has been associated with a reduced risk of advanced prostate cancer. Regular exercise can also help control weight and improve mood.[17]

Limit Calcium Intake:

- Some research suggests that high intake of calcium might be linked to an increased risk of prostate cancer, though more research is needed.[18]

Green Tea:

- Green tea has been researched for its potential to reduce the risk of advanced prostate cancer.[19]

Eat foods rich in Lycopene:

- Eat foods rich in lycopene, like watermelon and tomatoes. Lycopene is an antioxidant found to suppress the growth of prostate tissue and induce cell death in cells that need to be destroyed.[20]

Avoid Smoking:

- Smokers have an increased risk of dying from prostate cancer.[21]

---

[16] https://www.ncbi609

[17] https://www.ncbi.nlm.nih.gov/pmc/articles/PMC6527123/

[18] https://www.ncbi.nlm.nih.gov/pmc/articles/PMC6103569/

[19] https://academic.oup.com/aje/article/167/1/71/185454

[20] https://pubmed.ncbi.nlm.nih.gov/32768949/

[21] https://www.ncbi.nlm.nih.gov/pmc/articles/PMC9900478/

Regular Screening:

- Discuss with your healthcare provider what version of screening and/or surveillance is right for you.

Drink Coffee

- 16 prospective cohort studies were analyzed to conclude that a higher intake of coffee may be associated with a lower risk of prostate cancer.[22]

Have Sex

- Frequent ejaculation as a young adult has been linked to a decreased risk of developing prostate cancer. Two studies found that men who ejaculate 4.6-7 times a week were found to be 36% less likely to be diagnosed with prostate cancer before the age of 70.[23]

Why Awareness and Early Detection Matter

Establish a relationship with a primary care physician. Make sure he or she is interested in getting to know your family history, your medical history, and you as a whole. That is the best way to strategize for cancer prevention.

The Numbers: Studies indicate that the 5-year survival rate for localized prostate cancer (cancer confined to the prostate) is nearly 100%. However, this number drops significantly for cancers that have spread to distant parts of the body.

---

[22] https://bmjopen.bmj.com/content/11/2/e038902

[23] https://www.health.harvard.edu/mens-health/ejaculation_frequency_and_prostate_cancer

The Implication: Early detection of prostate cancer can make a world of difference. It not only increases the chances of successful treatment but can also reduce the intensity and duration of the treatment required.

Being Informed Means Being Empowered

Awareness is more than just knowing; it's about empowerment. A well-informed individual can:

1) *Make Better Choices*: From diet to lifestyle, an understanding of prostate health can guide men toward choices that bolster prostate well-being.

2) *Ask the Right Questions*: Awareness prepares men to engage in meaningful dialogues with their healthcare providers, ensuring they get the care they need.

3) *Break the Stigma*: Prostate issues, particularly those affecting sexual health, often come with undue embarrassment. Awareness can destigmatize these conversations, encouraging more men to come forward with their concerns.

Creating a Cascade Effect

When you become aware, you can become an advocate. Then, share your knowledge with friends, family, and your community.

CHAPTER 6:
THINGS TO MAKE SURE YOUR DOCTOR DOES

The truth is that I don't trust the healthcare system, and you likely do not either. You go to the doctor's office, and the physician barely has enough time to listen to you or really get to the root cause of the problem. So, instead of trying, he just pushes some pills your way and schedules you to come back to see how the medication helped. I've been a part of that system for years, and I have watched loved ones die as a result of this type of treatment.

So, in this section, I want to make sure you have all the tools and knowledge necessary to navigate through your doctor's visit in a way where you are the victor and not the victim. Victory can be yours! Here's how.

1) Go in with a smile and with 'suggestions.' The doctor is the gatekeeper to some tests you really do need. So don't piss him off and complicate things. Go in knowing that he thinks he is smarter than you, but go in knowing that he is wrong. Nobody knows your body better than you do.
2) Instead of demanding tests or asking questions that will make him look stupid or bruise his ego, tell him, 'I read something on the Mayo Clinic's website that suggested. . .' or 'My brother-in-law, who is a surgeon at Harvard Medical

Center said...' This will make him or her slow down, listen, and order whatever you suggest.

3) Never mention that you Googled anything, and don't mention that you saw anything on YouTube. They will instantly shut down and will no longer hear anything that you have to say.
4) Instead of letting him tell you your tests are normal, always ask for your own copies and to see the results.
5) Never agree to have a biopsy or any surgical procedure, even if they call it minor, without a second opinion.
6) Before getting a prostate biopsy, ask for an MRI. Sometimes, they try to just bundle the biopsy and MRI together. After you get the MRI, then you can get a second opinion.
7) If your doctor refuses to order an MRI, or your insurance won't pay for one, ask for an exosome prostate test to help determine if a prostate biopsy is really necessary.

The Cold Truth about Medical Exams

Navigating the medical landscape can sometimes feel like walking through a maze blindfolded, especially when it comes to prostate examinations.

Every prostate exam should begin with a physical exam. During the physical exam, the following should be completed for a prostate evaluation:

- A complete family history should be taken
- The doctor should ask questions about unintended weight loss, bowel habits, urinary symptoms, sexual activity
- Abdominal exam. Your physician should feel for bladder pain and loin pain.
- An examination of external genitals looking at the opening or the meatus of the penis
- Digital rectal exam (tenderness, size, shape, consistency, and lobes of the prostate)
- Urine dipstick (looking for an infection and protein leaking from the kidney)
- Sexually transmitted infection testing (STI testing)
- International Prostate Symptom Score - a questionnaire that speaks to symptom severity
- Kidney function blood tests
- PSA, male hormone panel (if you haven't already had one this year), and hs-crp (to measure inflammation in the body)

The PSA Controversy: The Prostate-Specific Antigen (PSA) test is a blood test predominantly used to screen for prostate cancer. The test's high false-positive rate means many men can undergo invasive and potentially unnecessary biopsies based solely on these results. While the PSA test remains a crucial tool, it's essential to approach it with informed caution.

Digital Rectal Examination (DRE): A mainstay in prostate check-ups, the DRE involves a healthcare professional using their finger to palpate the prostate through the rectal wall. It's designed to detect any abnormalities, like lumps or hard areas. The efficacy of this method, however, can vary wildly. Much depends on the practitioner's experience and skill. Some smaller tumors might go unnoticed, while benign conditions might be mistaken for something more sinister.

A Dual Approach for Better Insight: Leading urologists often recommend a combination of both the PSA test and the DRE. By doing both, doctors get a more complete picture.

Beyond the Basics: In the ever-evolving field of medicine, new diagnostic tools that promise more precision and less invasiveness are emerging. Advanced imaging techniques, biomarker tests, and genomics are here. Yet, they aren't standard everywhere. Why settle for the basics when the advanced might be within reach?

After you have been diagnosed with BPH, should the following tests be part of a complete evaluation?

- post-void residual checks to see how much urine stays stuck in your bladder
- urine flow studies - urodynamic studies to see how the bladder empties and fills
- PSA testing to help predict prostate volume or size if one hasn't been done yet
- Ultrasound of the urinary tract to look for residual urine, enlarged kidneys, and or enlarged ureters
- cystoscopy - a lighted camera tube that is about the size of a pencil is placed into the head of the penis to look inside the urethra and bladder.

Questions Your Doctor Doesn't Want to Hear

Your health journey is a partnership between you and your healthcare provider. By asking the right questions, you equip yourself with knowledge and signal to your doctor that you are an active participant in your care, eager to explore all avenues to achieve the best possible health outcomes.

Medical examinations can often feel one-sided. A doctor performs tests, asks questions, and provides insights or diagnoses. But as a patient, you're not just a passive participant. Here are some potentially uncomfortable—but crucial—questions you might consider posing during your next visit:

"What are the Limitations of These Tests?" No test is perfect. Whether it's the PSA test, DRE, or any other examination, each has its own set of limitations. Understanding these can help set realistic expectations and guide decisions about additional or alternative testing.

"Are There Newer or More Advanced Tests Available?" Medical science is ever-evolving. Sometimes, newer, more accurate tests are available but aren't part of standard protocols due to various reasons (e.g., cost, lack of awareness). It's essential to know all your options.

"What Would You Recommend If I Were Your Family Member?" This personalizes the question and may help in getting a candid response. Doctors often have insights into the nuances of treatment options that might not be immediately apparent to patients.

"Are There Any Lifestyle or Dietary Changes I Can Make to Improve My Prostate Health?" While medication and medical interventions have their place, lifestyle and dietary changes can often profoundly impact health. These modifications can be preventative and restorative.

"How Many Times Have You Performed This Procedure?" If surgery or a particular procedure is recommended, knowing your doctor's experience level can be reassuring. Experience often correlates with proficiency.

"What Are the Long-term Impacts of This Treatment?" Sometimes, treatments can have side effects or long-term implications that aren't immediately obvious. Knowing these can help in making an informed decision.

"Are There Any Alternative Treatments or Therapies Worth Considering?" Conventional treatments are not the only options. Sometimes, alternative or complementary therapies might offer benefits, especially when used in tandem with traditional methods.

Will my insurance cover an MRI of the prostate?

You said I need a biopsy. Can we do an MRI first?

Part II
Prostate Health: The Proactive Approach

In a world where the pressures of daily life often overshadow personal health priorities, being proactive about prostate health is not just commendable—it's critical. The prostate, a small yet influential gland, warrants this proactive approach for several reasons:

1) *Anticipation Over Reaction*: The early stages of many prostate issues may not manifest in clear symptoms. Rather than waiting for problems to arise and then reacting, proactive screening and attention can catch potential issues before they escalate. This anticipatory approach can save health complications and the emotional and financial tolls of advanced treatments.

2) *Consistent Monitoring*: One-off checks can provide snapshots of health, but consistent monitoring offers a movie reel, capturing the progression or regression of health over time. Regular check-ups allow you to set a baseline, making it easier to spot anomalies. It's like tracking your financial growth—just as you wouldn't check your bank account once and forget about it, your health, too, deserves consistent attention.

3) *Empowerment Through Knowledge*: Being proactive is synonymous with being informed. The more you know

about your prostate health, the better positioned you are to make decisions. This knowledge isn't just limited to medical facts; it encompasses understanding your body, recognizing changes, and feeling empowered to discuss concerns with healthcare professionals.

4) *Holistic Lifestyle Choices*: Proactivity extends beyond the doctor's office. Awareness of the prostate's role and its health implications can guide daily decisions—from what you eat and how often you exercise to how you manage stress. A proactive approach fosters a lifestyle that champions prostate well-being.

5) *Averting Potential Health Ripple Effects*: Prostate health doesn't operate in isolation. Issues like BPH or prostatitis can impact bladder health, kidney function, and overall quality of life. By being proactive about the prostate, you also take a stand for your broader health landscape.

CHAPTER 7:
LIFESTYLE, SEX, AND THE PROSTATE

Our lifestyle, including dietary choices, physical activity levels, and even stress management, plays a pivotal role in the overall health of the prostate. These elements not only impact the prostate's health directly but also influence sexual vitality, which is closely tied to prostate well-being.

The Importance of Exercise: More Than Just Cardio

It's a well-established fact that exercise is pivotal for overall health, but when it comes to the prostate, specific types of activities can offer targeted benefits:

Pelvic Floor Exercises: Often associated with women's health, especially post-pregnancy, pelvic floor exercises are equally essential for men. Strengthening the pelvic floor muscles can support the prostate and bladder, improving urinary continence. It can also enhance erectile function and orgasmic response, linking back to our earlier discussion on the prostate's role in sexual health.

Aerobic and Cardiovascular Exercise: Regular cardio, be it jogging, swimming, cycling, or even brisk walking, can improve blood flow throughout the body, including the pelvic region.

Enhanced circulation ensures the prostate receives the nutrients and oxygen required for optimal function. Furthermore, cardiovascular exercises can help in maintaining a healthy weight, which is linked to reduced risks of prostate issues.

Resistance Training: Strength training, especially exercises targeting the core and lower body, can benefit the prostate indirectly. A strong core supports the pelvic region, and leg exercises like squats can promote healthy blood flow to the pelvic organs.

Yoga and Stretching: The flexibility and relaxation benefits of yoga can be particularly beneficial for the pelvic region. Poses that focus on hip opening and pelvic relaxation can alleviate tension, promoting better blood flow and potentially aiding in toxin elimination from the prostate.

Stress Reduction through Exercise: Chronic stress can lead to hormonal imbalances, which might have implications for prostate health. Exercise acts as a natural stress reliever, releasing endorphins—the body's feel-good chemicals. Whether it's the tranquility of a gentle walk in nature or the rush after an intense workout, the stress-alleviating properties of exercise are undeniable.

The takeaway here is multifaceted: exercise isn't just about heart health or muscle building. For men, a well-rounded fitness regimen can have direct and indirect benefits for the prostate. Incorporating a mix of aerobic, resistance, flexibility, and pelvic-specific exercises can lay the foundation for robust prostate health and overall male vitality.

Foods and Ingredients Silently Wreaking Havoc on Your Prostate

While certain foods actively support prostate health, others may contribute to inflammation, hormonal imbalance, and other conditions that could spell trouble for the prostate. Being aware of these can help you make informed choices:

Processed Meats: Processed foods, especially processed meats like bacon, sausages, and hot dogs, often contain preservatives and other chemicals that might be harmful. Some studies suggest a link between high consumption of processed meats and an increased risk of prostate cancer.

Dairy Products: While the research is mixed, some studies indicate that high consumption of dairy, especially whole milk, might be associated with an increased risk of prostate cancer. The cause isn't entirely clear, but it might be related to the hormone content in dairy or its impact on certain growth factors. If you enjoy dairy, consider switching to goat's milk based products. If not, your dairy should be hormone-free, antibiotic-free, and organic.

Alcohol: Moderate alcohol consumption might be heart-healthy, but excessive drinking, especially binge drinking, can raise prostate cancer risk. It's always wise to consume alcohol in moderation.

Sugary Beverages and Snacks: High sugar consumption can lead to obesity, a known risk factor for prostate cancer. Moreover, constant sugar spikes can lead to insulin resistance, which has been linked to a higher risk of prostate and other cancers.

Trans Fats: Found in many processed foods, trans fats are known culprits for heart health. Their inflammatory properties might also impact the prostate, making checking food labels and minimizing their intake essential.

Caffeine: While moderate caffeine intake from sources like coffee has its benefits, excessive caffeine, especially from sugary energy drinks, might exacerbate urinary symptoms in men with BPH.

Calcium Supplements: While calcium is vital for bone health, some studies have linked excessive calcium supplementation to a higher risk of prostate cancer. It's always a good idea to get most of your nutrients, including calcium, from whole food sources.

When thinking about diet and prostate health, balance is the key. A diet rich in fruits, vegetables, whole grains, and lean proteins, coupled with awareness of potential problematic foods, sets the stage for optimal prostate health.

Stress, Sleep, and Their Silent Effects on Prostate Health

The modern world is bustling with challenges that can take a toll on our mental and emotional well-being. Stress and sleep deprivation, while seemingly unrelated to the prostate, can significantly impact its health in subtle yet profound ways.

The Hormonal Connection: Stress triggers the release of the hormone cortisol, often termed the "stress hormone." While cortisol is essential in short bursts (like in response to immediate threats), chronically elevated levels can disrupt the delicate balance of hormones in the body. Since the prostate's health is closely tied to male hormones, primarily testosterone, a sustained imbalance can have adverse effects on the gland.

Immune System and Stress: Chronic stress can weaken the immune system, making the body more susceptible to infections and diseases. A compromised immune system can increase the risk of prostatitis (inflammation of the prostate) and potentially affect the body's ability to fend off precancerous cells.

Sleep – The Natural Healer: Sleep is the time when the body repairs and regenerates. During the deep phases of sleep, cell repair and growth are accelerated. A lack of quality sleep can hamper this natural process, potentially leaving the prostate and other organs more vulnerable to issues.

Mental Well-being and Prostate Health: It's a two-way street. Chronic stress and sleep deprivation can lead to anxiety and depression. Conversely, concerns about prostate health, especially if one is diagnosed with a prostate condition, can further escalate stress levels. It's a cycle that underscores the importance of mental health in the broader spectrum of prostate well-being.

The Relaxation Response: Techniques such as meditation, deep breathing exercises, and even regular physical activity can elicit the body's relaxation response, a state of deep rest that can counteract the effects of stress. By regularly tapping into this state, one can effectively mitigate some of the adverse impacts of chronic stress on the prostate.

The silent warriors—stress and sleep—play pivotal roles in the overarching realm of prostate health. Recognizing their impact and adopting a proactive approach towards managing stress and ensuring quality sleep can be instrumental in maintaining a healthy prostate and overall well-being.

CHAPTER 8:
PROSTATE MASSAGE - A HIDDEN SECRET

The prostate is such an important aspect of erectile strength and power. Massage of the prostate has been used for centuries in physician's offices, holistic care centers, and at home to treat premature ejaculation, erectile dysfunction, prostate inflammation, and low semen production.

A famed prostate specialist, Dr. Lockhart, wrote in a medical journal published in 1919 that "the effect of massage on the prostate consists in emptying the pus pockets into the urethra, relieving the engorged blood vessels and lymphatics of the stroma, and liberating the reparative process by inducing a more liberal supply of fresh blood and lymph to the entire organ."

How Does Prostate Massage Work?

During the late 1800s, patients would often visit their physician's office 2-3 times a month to have the prostate massaged and milked of any substance present. This practice has been largely replaced by a class of medications called alpha-blockers.

Although there haven't been major scientific studies on prostate massage and ED, I will be one of the many physicians to stand by the statement that if prostate cancer and infection are not present, patients have stronger and better erections with regular prostate massage.

Although prostatic massage hasn't been studied in a major way, there is a scientific theory as to why prostate massage may help with:

- Help drain occluded ejaculatory ducts that have filled up over the years and decrease fibrosis (stiffness)

- Improve the flow of nutrient-rich blood to the prostate

- Stimulate the nerves and blood vessels (neurovascular bundle) that are responsible for an erection

- Remove stagnant fluids and potentially flush out built-up toxins

Stimulation of the prostate through massage has been theorized to:

1) Erectile Dysfunction
2) Prostate Enlargement
3) Prostatitis
4) Nocturia (nighttime urination)

Taoist philosophers and tantric teachers use prostate massage to maintain and promote extreme sexual conditioning. Some ancient rulers and elites received regular prostate massages from their staff to keep their stamina and erections in tip-top shape.

Disclaimer: Before you consider doing the prostatic massage, you have to consult your physician first and make sure that no cancer is present and that there isn't an existing infection. Prostate massage should not be done during a painful prostatitis flare-up or when there are active hemorrhoids present.

The prostate sits at the base of the penis, in front of the rectum, and right beneath the bladder.

If you massage your prostate too vigorously, you can cause damage to the lining of your rectum and may cause a flare-up or create the potential for hemorrhoids to develop. Make sure you are gentle with the prostate massage.

Also, If you have an infection, inflammation, or prostate cancer, a prostatic massage can potentially make all of these conditions worse. That is why it is extremely important that you consult with your physician first and that they do a complete prostate exam before you begin to regularly massage your prostate.

Dickups to Strengthen Your Pelvic Floor

A Dick-Up is a push-up for your D*.

Pelvic floor exercises have been popularized for women, but the same attention has not been placed on them for men. Nobody discusses the fact that without exercise, your pelvis will weaken, as will your erections. You will not be able to last as long, your ejaculate won't shoot out as it used to, and you will find that getting and keeping an erection may become difficult. The pelvic floor supports the bladder and the prostate. If it is weak and deconditioned, urinary symptoms will worsen over time.

Pelvic floor exercises can increase erectile function, decrease incontinence, and strengthen urinary sphincters. The bulbocavernosus muscle wraps around the base of the penis like a sling, and it has three very important jobs: 1) It applies pressure to the deep dorsal vein to make sure that blood does not escape during an erection and that your erection stays strong. 2) It contracts during ejaculation. 3) After you urinate, it helps you drain that last bit of urine out of your urethra. So, these exercises can help improve urine control and also strengthen your ability to ejaculate.

The Dickup

1) Find a comfortable place to relax. You need a place where you can have uninterrupted time for at least 15 min. Take deep breaths in and out and find your pelvic floor muscles by

doing the following: Pretend that you are trying to prevent gas from escaping from your anus. Find those muscles that you use and hold them in a clinched or contracted state. If you are having erection difficulty, these muscles are likely weakened, and it is normal to have trouble isolating them.

2) Now, practice your contractions. Focus on the muscles that you have isolated. Now contract them and hold them for 10 seconds. Then relax them for 3 seconds and repeat the cycle 3 more times. Breathe in while you contract, and breathe out while you release. Repeat this process while standing and then while lying down. Make this part of your daily routine. Either do it right before you get up in the morning or before you go to bed at night.

3) As you get stronger, switch it up and hold your contractions for as long as possible. Most men see results within 2-3 weeks of starting their daily Dick-Ups. Continue Dick-Ups a few times a week for the rest of your life.

CHAPTER 9:
DIET, SUPPLEMENTS, AND THEIR UNDERRATED IMPORTANCE

The Prostate-Boosting Foods Your Doctor Didn't Suggest

Diet plays a crucial role in every facet of our health, and the prostate is no exception. While certain foods are universally recognized for their prostate-friendly properties, some lesser-known foods and ingredients also offer compelling benefits. Here's a breakdown of some of the prostate-boosting foods that often fly under the radar:

Flaxseeds: Rich in omega-3 fatty acids and lignans, flaxseeds can help reduce prostate inflammation and might even play a role in preventing prostate cancer by inhibiting cancer cell growth.[24] It's best to consume them ground for maximum absorption.

Pomegranates: This ruby-red fruit has been the focus of numerous studies due to its high concentration of antioxidants. Pomegranate juice, in particular, has shown potential in slowing the progression of prostate cancer and improving PSA levels.[25]

---

[24] https://www.ncbi.nlm.nih.gov/pmc/articles/PMC3624628/

[25] https://www.mdpi.com/1422-0067/15/9/14949

Turmeric: Known for its anti-inflammatory properties, thanks to the active compound curcumin, turmeric might be beneficial in preventing prostate conditions and even slowing down the progression of existing prostate diseases.[26]

Green Tea: Rich in the polyphenol EGCG, green tea has shown promise in inhibiting the growth of cancer cells and reducing tumor growth, especially concerning prostate cancer. Studies seem to indicate that the more you drink, the more your risk decreases. Risk is significantly decreased with 7 cups/day. [27] There is also evidence that the ECGC in green tea can help reduce the overproduction of prostate cells, prevent the onset of BPH, and improve bladder emptying. Men with BPH took 500mg of green tea a day, and after six weeks, they showed improvement in quality of life, urine flow, and decreased inflammation.[28]

Cruciferous Vegetables: While broccoli and cauliflower are often recommended for their anticancer properties, lesser-known members of this family, like bok choy and Brussels sprouts, are equally potent. They contain sulforaphane, a compound believed to target cancer cells and reduce tumor size.[29]

Pumpkin Seeds: In a study of over 1400 men with BPH, 1 group ate 5g of pumpkin seeds and 1000mg of pumpkin seed extract daily

---

[26] https://www.ncbi.nlm.nih.gov/pmc/articles/PMC4618860/

[27] https://www.ncbi.nlm.nih.gov/pmc/articles/PMC5380255/

[28] https://www.ncbi.nlm.nih.gov/pmc/articles/PMC4003843/

[29] https://pubmed.ncbi.nlm.nih.gov/37343525/

for 12 months, and the other group was given a placebo. 58.5% of the men with BPH who ate the pumpkin seeds and took the extract had improved urinary symptoms, quality of life, and nighttime urination.[30]

Nuts: Nuts are rich in zinc and a healthy prostate will have a large store of zinc. When normal prostate tissue is compared to prostate cancer tissue, normal prostate tissue always has higher levels of zinc.[31]

While these foods provide myriad benefits, it's important to remember that no single food or ingredient is a magic bullet. A holistic, varied, and balanced diet, combined with other lifestyle factors, is the key to optimal prostate health.

Supplements: Nature's Answer to Prostate Vitality

While a balanced diet lays the foundation for prostate health, supplements can serve as additional support, filling in the gaps and addressing specific concerns. Here are some of the renowned supplements for prostate well-being:

Beta-Sitosterol: Found in various plants, beta-sitosterol is a supplement shown to relieve BPH symptoms. 200 patients with BPH were treated with 20mg of beta-sitosterol three times a day or

---

[30] https://pubmed.ncbi.nlm.nih.gov/25196580/

[31] https://www.ncbi.nlm.nih.gov/pmc/articles/PMC7424038/

given a placebo. After 6 months, the ones taking beta-sitosterol saw improvement in urine flow, less urine left over in the bladder, and significant improvement in symptoms.[32]

Saw Palmetto: One of the most well-known supplements for prostate health, Saw Palmetto has been used for decades to relieve symptoms associated with benign prostatic hyperplasia (BPH). It's believed to work by reducing the size of the inner lining of the prostate, which puts pressure on the tubes that carry urine.

Zinc: Zinc plays a crucial role in prostate health. The highest amount of zinc in the body is thought to be within the prostate gland. Some studies suggest that a zinc deficiency might be linked to certain prostate disorders. However, it is also important to note that more than 75mg of zinc per day over 15 years may increase the risk of aggressive forms of prostate cancer.[33]

Pygeum: Derived from the bark of the African cherry tree, pygeum has been traditionally used to treat urinary disorders. Modern research supports its benefits for reducing BPH symptoms.

Stinging Nettle: Often paired with saw palmetto in prostate supplements, stinging nettle root can help alleviate some of the symptoms of BPH, including reduced urinary flow.

---

[32] https://www.thelancet.com/journals/lancet/article/PIIS0140-6736(95)91085-9/fulltext

[33] https://link.springer.com/article/10.1007/s10654-022-00922-0

Omega-3 Fatty Acids: These essential fats, predominantly found in fish oil, have anti-inflammatory properties. While their direct impact on the prostate is still under study, their overall benefits for heart health and inflammation make them a valuable addition.

Pumpkin Seed Extract: Rich in phytosterols and omega-3s, pumpkin seeds have been traditionally used to support prostate health, especially in reducing symptoms of BPH.

Things To Remember

Consultation is Key: Before starting any supplement regimen, it's imperative to consult with a healthcare professional. Supplements can interact with medications or have side effects.

Purity and Source Matter: The supplement industry varies in quality. Ensure that any supplement you consider is from a reputable source, third-party tested for purity, and free from harmful contaminants.

Holistic Approach: Supplements should complement a balanced diet and healthy lifestyle, not replace them.

CHAPTER 10:
EVERYDAY PRODUCTS - THE HIDDEN ENEMIES

The modern world offers conveniences that were unimaginable a few decades ago. However, some of these conveniences come at a cost. There are chemicals and substances present in daily products that, unbeknownst to many, might have implications for prostate health.

The Hormonal Imbalance Conspiracy: Fact or Fiction?

In recent years, a growing number of voices have sounded the alarm about potential threats to male hormonal balance. With increasing reports of chemicals and substances in daily products that can mimic or inhibit hormones, some have started to question whether there's a broader agenda or conspiracy at play. Is the modern environment deliberately structured to undermine male health, particularly the prostate? Let's break down the facts.

Endocrine Disruptors: At the center of this discussion are endocrine disruptors. These are chemicals that can interfere with the endocrine system, which produces hormones regulating a wide array of body functions. These are everywhere. Examples include BPA, phthalates, and certain pesticides. They can mimic, block, or alter hormone behavior in the body. There's a growing body of evidence that suggests prolonged exposure to endocrine disruptors may increase the risk of developing hormone-related cancers, including prostate cancer.

Unintended Consequences: It's essential to understand that many of these chemicals were introduced into consumer products because of their functional properties. BPA, for instance, makes plastics more durable. Phthalates can enhance the flexibility of plastics. Their potential health implications might not have been fully understood when they were first incorporated into products.

Regulatory Challenges: With thousands of chemicals in use and new ones being introduced, regulators face a monumental task in assessing and managing potential health risks. While some countries have been proactive in limiting or banning substances known to be harmful, others lag behind, leading to uneven protection levels for consumers worldwide.

The Plausible Connection: While a grand conspiracy to deliberately harm male health is unlikely, the cumulative effect of various endocrine disruptors and other harmful chemicals in our environment cannot be dismissed. Hormonal imbalances can indeed affect prostate health, along with other aspects of male health.

Empowerment through Knowledge: Rather than getting lost in conspiracy theories, the best approach is to arm oneself with knowledge. One can reduce risk and support their overall health by understanding the potential threats and taking proactive steps, like opting for BPA-free products or using organic produce.

In conclusion, while it's improbable that there's a deliberate conspiracy to undermine male health, the unintentional consequences of our modern lifestyle and environment are clear. Awareness and informed choices are our best defenses against potential threats to prostate health.

Chemical Culprits in Everyday Products

Our modern environment is a double-edged sword. While innovations have undoubtedly improved our quality of life in many ways, they've also introduced a slew of chemicals into our daily routines, some of which could have implications for prostate health. Here's a closer look:

Triclosan: Often found in antibacterial soaps and some toothpastes, triclosan can act as an endocrine disruptor. Its long-term effects on the human body are still being studied, but it's worth noting that the FDA has raised concerns about its widespread use.

Phthalates:

Polychlorinated Biphenyls (PCBs): These industrial chemicals, banned in many countries, still linger in the environment and can accumulate in our bodies. Some research links PCBs to an increased risk of prostate cancer.

Perfluorinated Chemicals (PFCs): Used to make products resistant to water, grease, or stains, PFCs can be found in everything from non-stick cookware to water-repellent clothing. Some studies suggest that they can interfere with hormone function.

Artificial Fragrances: Synthetic fragrances in personal care products, air fresheners, and detergents often contain phthalates. As we've already discussed, phthalates are potential endocrine disruptors that can have implications for prostate health.

Arsenic: This heavy metal can contaminate drinking water, particularly in certain regions. Chronic exposure to arsenic has been linked to various health issues, including an increased risk of prostate cancer.

Toxins in Food and Everyday Products: Impact on Prostate Health

The Toxic Assault on the Prostate

Every day, we are bombarded by an array of chemicals and toxins that are omnipresent in our food and everyday products. From the pesticides sprayed on our produce to the parabens and phthalates in our personal care items, these substances can disrupt the delicate hormonal balance within the body and have been implicated in the development of various health issues, including prostate cancer.

Prostate Perpetrators

1) Pesticides and Herbicides: Used in conventional farming, many of these substances mimic estrogen, a hormone that, in excess, can fuel the growth of certain types of prostate cancer cells. Organochlorides, a class of chemicals once found in pesticides like DDT, can linger in the environment and accumulate in the food chain, posing risks to prostate health.

2) BPA (Bisphenol A): Found in plastic containers and linings of canned foods, BPA is a known endocrine disruptor that can mimic the body's hormones and interfere with the production, secretion, transport, action, function, and elimination of natural hormones.

3) Phthalates: These chemicals, used to make plastics more flexible, are found in various products, including food packaging, and can disrupt the endocrine system. Studies have suggested a link between phthalate exposure and increased risk of prostate cancer.

4) Heavy Metals: Cadmium and arsenic, contaminants found in some foods and water supplies, have been associated with an increased risk of prostate cancer due to their carcinogenic and estrogen-mimicking properties.

5) Artificial Hormones: Hormones given to livestock to promote growth can enter the human body through meat and dairy consumption, potentially impacting hormone balance and prostate health.

Sidestep the Toxin Trap

1) Choose Organic: Opt for organic produce to minimize exposure to harmful pesticides and herbicides. Organic certification prohibits the use of most synthetic pesticides and fertilizers.

2) BPA-Free Products: Select BPA-free plastics and cans. Better yet, use glass or stainless-steel containers to store food and beverages.

3) Mindful Meat Consumption: Eat less meat, and when you do, choose organic and grass-fed options to reduce the intake of artificial hormones and antibiotics.

4) Filter Your Water: Use a high-quality water filter that can remove heavy metals and other contaminants from your drinking water.

5) Natural Personal Care: Look for personal care products that are free from parabens, phthalates, and other harmful chemicals. The Environmental Working Group's (EWG) Skin Deep database can be a valuable resource for identifying safer products.

6) Detoxifying Diet: Incorporate foods known for their detoxifying properties, such as cruciferous vegetables (e.g., broccoli, cauliflower), which can help in the elimination of harmful estrogens and other toxins from the body.

7) Household Cleaners: Use natural cleaning products or make your own from ingredients like vinegar, baking soda, and essential oils to reduce exposure to environmental toxins.

By adopting these strategies, we can reduce our toxic burden and potentially lower the risk of prostate issues, including cancer. Emphasizing prevention through a clean and conscious lifestyle is paramount to maintaining prostate health and overall well-being.

The takeaway is pretty clear. We've got to be on the lookout for these chemicals that are hidden in so many everyday products. By doing that, we're not just protecting our overall health; we're also making sure that our prostate stays the right size, which keeps us peeing without trouble and maintaining a good sex life. It's all about being smart, staying informed, and choosing the right stuff to keep our bodies running smoothly.

Prostate Health for Peak Performance

Most men aren't aware of the profound connection between their prostate health and their sexual performance. This walnut-sized gland, situated just below the bladder, plays a pivotal role in the male sexual response. Here's why taking care of it can significantly enhance your intimate moments:

1) **Central Role in Pleasure:** The prostate is sometimes referred to as the "male G-spot." When stimulated, either directly during specific activities or indirectly during other forms of arousal, it can produce intense pleasure. An unhealthy prostate, on the other hand, might reduce sensitivity or even cause discomfort.

2) **Ejaculation and Fluid Production:** The prostate produces seminal fluid, a major component of ejaculation. This fluid nourishes and protects the sperm, ensuring its viability for fertilization. A healthy prostate ensures the proper volume and quality of this fluid, which can influence the intensity of the male orgasm.

3) **Erection Quality:** While the prostate isn't directly responsible for erections, its health can influence erection quality. Prostatitis, inflammation of the prostate, or other prostate issues can impede blood flow or cause discomfort, leading to challenges in maintaining a firm erection.

4) **Endocrine Connection:** The prostate is affected by male hormones, primarily testosterone. A balanced hormonal profile, which can be influenced by diet, exercise, and other lifestyle factors, supports prostate health. And as we know, testosterone plays a significant role in male libido and sexual responsiveness.

5) **Confidence and Mental Well-being:** It's not just about the physiological. Knowing that your prostate is in good health can bolster confidence in intimate situations. Worrying about potential discomfort or the implications of an unhealthy prostate can introduce mental barriers to peak sexual performance.

To harness the full potential of one's sexual health, focusing on the prostate is indispensable.

The Power of Knowledge: Taking Charge of Your Prostate Health

The prostate, while a small gland, plays an essential role in a man's life, affecting everything from sexual pleasure to fertility. And yet, it remains a misunderstood and often neglected organ.

Recognize and accept the vital role the prostate plays. It's not just about disease prevention; it's about optimizing function and ensuring a high quality of life.

Staying Updated: With medical research and studies being updated constantly, keeping abreast of the latest findings is crucial. This doesn't mean following every new fad but understanding the core principles of prostate health and how they evolve.

Being Proactive: As with many health issues, prevention is often more effective than treatment. Regular check-ups, a balanced diet, and a lifestyle that prioritizes well-being can all contribute to optimal prostate health.

Create Your Personal Prostate Care Plan

Take on a Tailored Approach: Everyone's body is different. While general guidelines are beneficial, understanding your unique risk factors and needs is vital. Genetics, lifestyle, and past medical history all play a role.

Consult with Professionals Who Respect You & Your Knowledge: Despite the vast amount of information available online, personal consultations with a healthcare professional remain invaluable. They can help fine-tune your care plan.

Prostate care isn't just about the prostate. It's about overall health. Ensuring cardiovascular health, mental well-being, and hormonal balance all play a role in keeping your prostate healthy.

Advocate for Comprehensive Prostate Care

Speak Up: The more people talk about prostate health, the more attention it will garner from the medical community and policymakers. Share your knowledge with others and help break the taboos surrounding the topic.

Support Research: Whether it's through donations, participation in studies, or simply staying informed, supporting prostate health research can lead to breakthroughs that benefit everyone.

Community Involvement: Joining prostate health groups, participating in awareness events, and advocating for better healthcare policies can make a significant difference. Together, voices are louder and more influential.

In conclusion, prostate health, like all aspects of our well-being, requires vigilance, education, and proactive action. With the knowledge and tools at our disposal, every man has the power to optimize his prostate health and ensure a fulfilling, vibrant life.

Made in USA - North Chelmsford, MA
49908_9798868103025
12.26.2023 2121